BI 3277140 1

PIHLM

D0774767

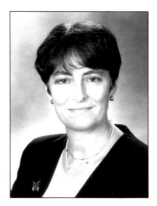

Angela Coulter is Chief Executive of Picker Institute Europe. A UK-registered charity, with its headquarters in Oxford, England and offices in Germany, Sweden and Switzerland, the Picker Institute works with European health care providers to obtain feedback from patients and promote patient-centred care.

A social scientist by training, Angela has a doctorate in health services research from the University of London and has published widely on a variety of topics. She is Visiting Professor in Health Services Research at the University of Oxford, Visiting Fellow at Nuffield College, Oxford, a Governor of Oxford Brookes University and an Honorary Fellow of the Faculty of Public Health Medicine. From 1993–99 Angela was an Executive Director of the King's Fund in London leading their work on health policy analysis, research and service development. Prior to that she worked for 12 years at the University of Oxford where she established and directed the Health Services Research Unit.

Angela is currently a member of the European Commission's G10 High Level Group on Innovation and Provision of Medicines; a member of the Department of Health's Quality Task Force and Medicines Partnership Task Force; and an advisor to WHO on responsiveness surveys. She is the founding editor of *Health Expectations*, an international peer-reviewed journal of public participation in health care and health policy. Her other books include *Hospital Referrals* (with Martin Roland), Oxford University Press 1992; *Informing Patients* (with Vikki Entwistle and David Gilbert), King's Fund 1998; *The Global Challenge of Health Care Rationing* (with Chris Ham), Open University Press 2000; and *The European Patient of the Future* (with Helen Magee), Open University Press, forthcoming.

The Autonomous Patient

Ending paternalism in medical care

TSO

Published by TSO (The Stationery Office) and available from:

Online
www.tso.co.uk/bookshop

Mail, Telephone, Fax & E-mail
TSO
PO Box 29, Norwich, NR3 1GN
Telephone orders/General enquiries: 0870 600 5522
Fax orders: 0870 600 5533
E-mail: book.orders@tso.co.uk
Textphone 0870 240 3701

TSO Shops
123 Kingsway, London, WC2B 6PQ
020 7242 6393 Fax 020 7242 6394
68-69 Bull Street, Birmingham B4 6AD
0121 236 9696 Fax 0121 236 9699
9-21 Princess Street, Manchester M60 8AS
0161 834 7201 Fax 0161 833 0634
16 Arthur Street, Belfast BT1 4GD
028 9023 8451 Fax 028 9023 5401
18-19 High Street, Cardiff CF10 1PT
029 2039 5548 Fax 029 2038 4347
71 Lothian Road, Edinburgh EH3 9AZ
0870 606 5566 Fax 0870 606 5588

TSO Accredited Agents
(see Yellow Pages)

and through good booksellers

© Nuffield Trust 2002
Third impression 2003
Applications for reproduction should be made to
The Nuffield Trust
59, New Cavendish Street,
London, W1M 7RD

ISBN 0 11 703056 2

Printed in the United Kingdom for The Stationery Office
161373 C5 12/03 916390

The Autonomous Patient

Ending paternalism in medical care

Angela Coulter, PhD

Chief Executive
Picker Institute Europe
and
Visiting Professor in Health Services Research
University of Oxford

The John Fry Fellowship, 2002

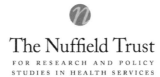

The Nuffield Trust

FOR RESEARCH AND POLICY
STUDIES IN HEALTH SERVICES

London: TSO

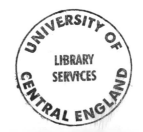

UNIVERSITY OF
LIBRARY
SERVICES
CENTRAL ENGLAND

ACKNOWLEDGEMENTS

This work would not have been possible without the help of the many researchers with whom I have collaborated on various studies of patients' views and experiences, my colleagues past and present at Picker Institute Europe, the King's Fund and the University of Oxford, and Paddy, Rachel and Alice Coulter who supported it in so many ways.

I am also grateful to the Editor of the British Medical Journal for permission to reproduce parts of my article 'After Bristol: putting patients at the centre' which appeared in BMJ 2002; 324: 648–5. This monograph aims to put flesh on the bones of the argument which first appeared in that article.

Above all I am indebted to the Trustees and staff of the Nuffield Trust for awarding me the John Fry Fellowship and for their support in the production of this book.

UNIVERSITY OF
CENTRAL ENGLAND

Book no. 32771401

Subject no. 362.1042 SAut

LIBRARY SERVICES

This work has been supported by the Nuffield Trust.

Contents

Preface

John Fry was one of the founding fathers of modern general practice. His extraordinary energy and commitment enabled him to combine the demanding roles of dedicated family doctor and insightful researcher. His meticulous documentation of the diseases experienced by patients in his practice in Beckenham, Kent, and his prolific output of publications describing the key roles of the GP, the primary care team and the context in which they worked, helped to define the role of the primary care doctor internationally and contributed to the growth and confidence of a profession which justifiably claims credit for the relative efficiency and effectiveness of the British NHS. It is therefore entirely appropriate that previous holders of the Nuffield Trust's John Fry Fellowship have all been GPs. My distinguished predecessors – David Morrell, John Hasler, Iona Heath, John Howie – have made significant contributions to what John Fry described as the transformation of British general practice "from a cottage industry to a well organised and confident branch of the medical profession".[1] For the most part they used their Fellowship lectures to focus on the changing roles and responsibilities of primary care professionals.

I am not a GP, nor am I medically trained, and my career has taken me beyond the confines of a single academic discipline. I prefer to describe myself as a health services researcher, which in my case can be translated as a sort of disciplinary hybrid – part medical sociologist, part epidemiologist, part health policy analyst, part educationalist, part specialist in development and change. With this mixed bag of skills I have spent the past 20 years observing health care in Britain (and elsewhere), trying to draw attention to its deficiencies and strengths. My task now is to turn the spotlight onto patients. In this monograph I shall argue that the role of the primary care professional needs further adaptation to accommodate the changing expectations of patients in the 21st century.

What then are my qualifications for attempting to articulate the patient's perspective? My career in health services research began in 1983 at the Department of Public Health and Primary Care at the University of Oxford, where I was responsible for a variety of studies including health behaviours and prevention in primary care, variations in surgical rates and in GP referral rates, development and use of information systems in primary care, women's health, techniques for quality improvement, the effects of the 1991 NHS reforms and the impact of treatments on patients' quality of life. I learnt a great deal during these ten years at the Oxford medical school where I was privileged to work alongside some of the leading experts in epidemiology and health services research, but in particular it left me with a healthy scepticism about over-optimistic claims of benefit from medical interventions and a sense that the patient's perspective was often left out of the equation.

A move to the King's Fund in 1993 enabled me to escape the drudgery of data collection for a while and to focus on the development and implementation of health care policy. There we concentrated our efforts on the extent to which government health policy made, or could make, a real impact on the experience of users of the health service. Once again I was struck by the gap between the policy rhetoric and the reality as experienced by patients and a strong feeling that there was a need to refocus on the everyday experience of patients and their interactions with the health system. When in 2000 I was offered the chance to go back to Oxford to lead the Picker Institute's efforts to promote patient-centred care in Europe, I was handed a wonderful opportunity, and a daunting responsibility, to try to make a reality out of my own rhetoric.

Picker Institute Europe is a small independent research and educational charity with very ambitious aims, namely to improve the quality of health care throughout Europe by enabling health care providers to view their services 'through the patient's eyes'. The origins of the organisation lie in the pioneering work of American academics, in particular Tom Delbanco and Paul Cleary at Harvard Medical School, and their colleague Susan Edgman-Levitan, President of the Picker Institute in Boston. Their work, and ours, was made possible by generous support from Harvey Picker and the Commonwealth Fund of New York, who had the vision to see that patient-centred care was an idea worth supporting. The founders of the Picker Institute focused their efforts on developing techniques for systematically measuring patients' experience of health care so as to identify problems and prioritise topics for quality improvement. But diagnosis, though necessary, is not sufficient, so we aim to go further than that. Our research tries to identify the most effective means of changing the system to ensure that patients' needs and preferences are truly centre stage in health care delivery and we constantly look for ways to keep these issues high up on the policy agenda.

In September 1999 the British Medical Journal (BMJ) published a special theme issue entitled 'Embracing patient partnership'. Following its publication visitors to the BMJ's website were asked to respond to a brief questionnaire asking their views on consulting styles (BMJ 16/10/99). The survey ran over a two-week period from 17 September to 4 October. The results are shown in Table 1 below.

TABLE 1

Responses to BMJ questionnaire on consultation styles[1]

	Doctor decides	*Doctor and patient decide together*	*Patient decides*
As a patient, which consulting style do you prefer?	56 (6.6%)	737 (87.0%)	54 (6.4%)
Which consulting style predominates today?	503 (59.6%)	298 (35.3%)	43 (5.1%)
Which consulting style do you think will predominate in 10 years' time?	75 (8.9%)	546 (64.7%)	223 (26.4%)

http://www.bmj.com/ 24th October 1999

Visitors to the BMJ website are certainly not representative of the general population. Predominantly medically trained professionals, they constitute a particularly well-informed and influential group. It is not particularly surprising, therefore, that respondents to this survey indicated a preference for a participative role in decisions about their own care, but the disjunction between the way in which they said they wanted to be treated when they were patients and their views of how most other patients are treated currently, was striking. Even more noteworthy was their sense that paternalistic consultation styles are on the way out, to be replaced by shared decision making or informed choice as the dominant modes.

If these survey respondents are correct, the next ten years will see a profound change in relationships between health professionals and their patients. The factors driving the change include rising educational standards, improvements in public access to health information and a decline in deference to professional authority. Government action has fuelled the change. Consumerism has been promoted as a central plank of health policy in many countries in the belief that consumer pressure and competition would drive up quality standards and increase value for money. But costs have continued to rise and there has been an upward trend in the number of complaints and law suits by dissatisfied patients, suggesting either that services have got worse or, more plausibly, that people are now more likely to seek redress when things go wrong. What are the implications of this change in public expectations of health services? What opportunities and challenges will this pose for those working in primary care?

This monograph argues that paternalism, which is still the defining characteristic of medical care in the British NHS and in the health systems of many other countries, has had its day. Instead we must redefine the patient's role to emphasise autonomy, emancipation and self-reliance rather than passivity and dependence. No longer is he or she simply a victim of illness. In the 21st century patients must be treated as co-producers of their own health and care-managers when they are ill. They must be encouraged to see themselves as decision-makers, evaluators, and stakeholders with a key role in shaping health policy. Health professionals must adapt their behaviour to accommodate this more active role. Developing and extending active partnerships with patients is the only way to ensure the sustainability of publicly-funded health care.

REFERENCE

[1]   Fry J. General practice and primary health care 1940s–1980s. London: Nuffield Provincial Hospitals Trust, 1988.

1. The case for change

"The quality of healthcare would be enhanced by a greater degree of respect and honesty in the relationship between healthcare professional and patient." [1]

Bristol Royal Infirmary Inquiry. Learning from Bristol. 2001

Evidence of sub-standard care

The scandal surrounding the excess death rate among children undergoing heart surgery at the Bristol Royal Infirmary during the 1980s and early 1990s was a defining moment in the history of the NHS. The subsequent public inquiry pointed to the manifest good intentions and long hours of dedicated work by the health care professionals involved, but placed the blame on *"a combination of circumstances which owed as much to general failings in the NHS at the time than to any individual failing."* [1] These failings included poor leadership, disorganisation, lack of transparency and an unhealthy 'club culture' among senior doctors.

In particular, Professor Ian Kennedy's Inquiry Team identified the need for substantial change in the way in which health professionals interact with patients and their carers. They made 198 recommendations, pre-eminent amongst which were exhortations to involve patients (or their parents) in decisions, to keep them informed, to improve communication with them, to provide them with counselling and support, to gain their informed consent for all procedures and processes, to elicit feedback and listen to their views, to be open and candid when adverse events occur, and to offer them opportunities to get involved in the planning, organisation and delivery of health care.

Improving responsiveness to patients has been a goal of health policy in the UK for several decades, but up to now most initiatives in this area have failed to make a noticeable difference to the everyday experience of most NHS patients. The harsh realities of budgetary pressures, staff shortages and other managerial imperatives tend to displace good intentions about informing and involving patients, responding quickly and effectively to their needs and wishes, and ensuring that they are treated in a dignified and supportive manner. This is the essence of patient-centred care and most health professionals strive to achieve it, but many clinical staff feel that the demands on them to improve efficiency and productivity have had a detrimental effect on their capacity to offer their patients the time and empathy that they need and hope for.[2]

There is a new urgency in the air now, though, and improving the patient's experience has been placed much higher up the agenda. In reaction to quality failures such as those in Bristol, the British government made patient-centredness the central theme in its NHS Plan, announcing a realignment of incentive systems to encourage improvements in performance, with patient feedback incorporated into the new star rating system for performance indicators.[3] This resort to carrot and stick may be necessary to kick start the move towards greater responsiveness to patients, but there are deeper reasons why health care providers ought to be moving in this direction.

There is almost universal agreement that the goals of a modern health system must include catering for patients' needs and expectations by providing equitable access to appropriate, effective, safe and efficient care which conforms to the highest quality standards and is accountable to those who pay for it. The manner in which care was delivered in Bristol and in many other hard-pressed corners of the NHS seems a long way from attainment of these goals. My contention is that they will not be achieved until those working in the NHS adopt a radically different view of the patients' role. There has been much talk of the need for a 'culture change' in the NHS, but little clarity about what needs changing and how to do it. This monograph outlines my view of what has gone wrong and what can be done about it. The problems are briefly outlined below. Supporting evidence and possible solutions are discussed in the following chapters.

Meeting expectations
It has become a cliché to remark that public expectations are rising faster than the ability of health services to meet them, but it remains one of the most important ironies of modern health care. At a time when expenditure on health care is increasing much faster than inflation in most countries and effective treatments are more widely available than ever before, there is evidence of growing public pessimism about the future of health systems.[4]

What has caused this crisis of confidence? Are people simply hoping for too much? Is this the inevitable result of over-selling the benefits of medical care, with disillusionment the inevitable consequence of allowing false hopes to persist? Or does the problem lie not in unrealistic public expectations, but in the failure of the health service to respond adequately to the needs of those who use it?

In a democracy the system for collective provision of health care requires continuing support from its citizens or electorate. The British public continues to provide strong support for the principle of taxation-funded health care, but memories of the fragmented and inequitable system that preceded its introduction are fading and the NHS can no longer trade on people's gratitude. Tolerance of long waiting times, lack of information, uncommunicative staff, and failure to seek patients' views and take account of their preferences is wearing thin. Politicians recognise this, hence their desire to modernise the system by encouraging greater responsiveness to patients. In the long run the survival of the NHS will depend on the extent to which this goal can be achieved.

Treatment choices
Information and involvement is at the heart of the patient-centred approach. If clinicians are ignorant of patients' values and preferences, patients may receive treatment which is inappropriate to their needs. Unfortunately there is evidence that clinicians sometimes fail to understand patients' preferences and patients aren't given the opportunity to play a full part in decisions about their care. Untested assumptions about what the patient wants can lead to unnecessary treatment. Informed consent procedures frequently fall short of the ideal, often relegated to hasty discussions with junior doctors whose main goal is to obtain a signature on a form. In this situation options and alternatives aren't discussed and the 'consent' implied by the signature cannot be said to be truly informed.

Failure to provide full and balanced information about risks and uncertainties can give rise to unrealistic expectations which in turn may be a cause of rising litigation rates. Patients are frequently given a biased and highly optimistic picture of the benefits of medical care. This can lead to unrealistic demands and disillusion. If patients are encouraged to believe there is an effective pill for every ill, or that surgery is risk-free, it is no wonder that they sometimes find the reality disappointing. There is a tendency to treat patients like children who need to be told what to do and reassured, instead of as responsible adults capable of assimilating information and using it to make informed choices. Misplaced paternalism which tries to "protect" patients from the bad news merely fuels false hopes and does no one – patients or clinicians – any good in the long run.

Managing care

The majority of health care is self-managed. People do not usually consult a health professional the minute they feel a bit under the weather. Most of us try first of all to help ourselves, often consulting family and friends in the process. There is a wealth of lay knowledge about illness and how to treat it, but this is often ignored or dismissed by health professionals.

Too often the way in which clinicians and patients interact tends to promote passivity and dependence instead of self-reliance, sapping self-confidence and undermining people's ability to cope. The patient's input is essential to defining and understanding the problem, identifying possible solutions and managing the illness, but their part in the diagnostic and healing process is rarely acknowledged. Patients' role in caring for themselves needs to be strengthened instead of being undermined. Poor communication and failure to take account of the patient's perspective is at the heart of the vast majority of formal complaints and legal actions. Many medical errors and adverse events might be avoided if patients were more actively engaged in their care.

Performance assessment and quality improvement

If we want to centre quality improvement efforts on the needs and wishes of patients, we must first understand how things look through their eyes and those of their carers. Receipt of regular feedback from patients on how they felt about the care they experienced has long been considered important in systems based on market competition, such as the American one, but up to now this aspect of quality assessment has been largely ignored in the NHS. Interest in patient feedback is beginning to grow, but many clinicians still see it as irrelevant, misleading or threatening. The idea that patients could make reliable assessments of their clinical care is often dismissed on the grounds that they are not qualified to judge its technical quality. That may be true, but the patient's experience of receiving care is an important part of quality assessment and deserves to be taken more seriously. This is much more than concerns about food or car parking. 'Hotel' facilities are part of the experience but most patients give much higher priority to relations with the clinicians treating them. Their views on interpersonal care should be systematically monitored to establish whether they are receiving care of optimal quality.

Patients have a legitimate and important role as evaluators of health care, both in generating reports on their own experience and in analysing and using information on the quality of care to make comparisons between health care providers and to inform their own choices. Up to now choice has not been a central value of the NHS, but lack of choice now looks like its Achilles heel. We expect to be able to make informed choices in most other aspects of our lives and there are signs of growing frustration with the lack of choice in health care. Increasing opportunities for choice in health care is a central plank of the government's modernisation project, but achieving this while maintaining the emphasis on the other central goal of equality of access will be a difficult task.

Public participation and accountability

One of the central principles of the NHS, still strongly subscribed to by most of those who use it, is the notion that health care should be equitably distributed according to need and not the ability to pay. Evidence of inequity, for example so-called postcode prescribing, is especially problematic because it strikes at the heart of what most people believe to be the core value of the NHS. The increasing gap between public expectations and the supply of services has led governments to consider new ways to ensure that limited resources are used efficiently and equitably. The establishment of the National Institute for Clinical Excellence (NICE) was an important step in the right direction, but it has tried to promote a purely technical approach to the problem and has sought to avoid discussion about values or rationing.[5]

In the past politicians have been reluctant to spell out for members of the public the financial consequences of their demands for health care. They preferred to propagate the idea that all demands could be met if only efficiency could be increased. Few were fooled, but despite several attempts to promote a more informed public debate, little was done to engage the public in serious discussion about priorities.[6] Recently it has been announced that NICE will set up a Citizen's Council to engage members of the public in thinking through the issues.[3] Perhaps the nettle is at last about to be grasped – we can only wait and see.

Redefining the patient's role

It's time to redefine the patient's role. No longer is he or she simply a passive victim of illness. In the 21st century the patient is a decision-maker, care manager and co-producer of health, an evaluator, a potential change agent, a taxpayer and an active citizen whose voice must be heard by decision-makers. Acknowledging these roles and developing and extending active partnerships with patients has become essential for all health care providers, and in particular for those working on the front-line in primary care.

The key to restoring confidence lies as much in the hands of clinicians as it does in politicians. Clinicians could do a great deal to help inform and educate those who seek their help. If the public can be helped to understand the limits of medical care as well as its potential benefits, they are much more likely to use health services appropriately and responsibly. Recognition of the patient as an active, autonomous player in the health care system should have profound consequences for the way in which health care is delivered. Relationships between health professionals and the public they serve need to be transformed at all levels, organisational as well as individual. Simply grafting on some new organisational structures to promote patient involvement or inviting a few lay people to sit on committees will not be sufficient. Much more fundamental change is required in the way in which patients and professionals interact. Managers and clinicians will have to be prepared to cede some power and patients must be willing to take greater responsibility for their own health. These changes are necessary to ensure the sustainability of collective health care provision.

Patient, client, consumer or user?

Before addressing these issues in more detail, I must explain, and perhaps defend, my use of terminology. To some, the idea that a patient could be autonomous (*"free to determine one's own actions"*, *"independent of others"*) will seem a contradiction in terms.[7] After all, the latin root of patient is patiens, *"one who suffers"*. Collins Dictionary provides a fairly neutral definition: *"a person who is receiving medical care"*. In itself this need not imply suffering or dependence or passivity, but our view of the word and the role it describes, is coloured by its other meanings, viz. *"enduring trying circumstances with even temper"*, *"tolerant, understanding"*, and, especially pertinent in the case of NHS patients, *"capable of accepting delay with equanimity"*!

Some have argued that the term *patient* should be dropped because it underlines the inferior status of recipients of health care.[8;9] If we were to call them something else, what should it be? None of the suggested alternatives is entirely satisfactory.

Client has been adopted by social workers, accountants, lawyers and other professionals but its Latin root, *cliens*, means *"one who is obliged to make supplications to a powerful figure for material assistance"*. Nowadays we think of clients for the most part as people who pay a professional to receive a service, but there is still a sense of subservience implied in the use of this term.

Consumer suggests both a financial relationship (a purchaser) and a particular political stance, implying that public services operate like commercial markets. Certainly people who use health services bring with them expectations which are influenced by their involvement as consumers of goods and services, and I have argued above that the health service needs to accommodate consumer values, such as the ability to make informed choices. As purchasers of services, consumers have some power over providers who have a vested interest in responding to their needs. For this reason some organised groups prefer this term, but others reject it on the grounds that consumerism is an individualistic concept which fails to capture the collectivist essence of health systems.

The term *user* is becoming popular among professionals in NHS circles and among some groups representing people with long-term medical conditions and those with mental health problems, but it is a clumsy word that implies a relationship with an inanimate object rather than an active partnership with care providers. It also carries connotations of drug misuse and can therefore be easily misunderstood.

The case for a change of terminology is unconvincing on several counts. If patients are accorded inferior status by health professionals, it seems unlikely that semantic change would be sufficient to achieve a change in their status. And, as Tallis has observed, none of the suggested alternatives encompasses notions of compassion and trust, essential components of an effective and satisfactory relationship when people are ill and vulnerable.[10] More importantly, there is little evidence that ill people object to the label 'patient'. For example, a survey of 147 people attending the psychiatric outpatient department of an inner-city teaching hospital found that 77% preferred to be called 'patient' rather than 'client' and only 14% disliked the term.[11]

The term *patient* will therefore be used in this monograph to describe people in receipt of medical care, both because it seems to be more acceptable than the alternatives to those who carry the label, and because it is the most widely understood term.

Autonomy

In their discussion of the ethical principle of autonomy, Beauchamp and Childress argue that it involves the ability to act intentionally, with understanding and free from controlling influences.[12] For the clinician to respect the patient's autonomy he/she must, at minimum, acknowledge their right to hold views, to make choices, and to take actions based on personal values and beliefs. This requires more than just non-interference or acquiescence with the patient's choices. They argue that the clinician has an obligation to build up or maintain the patient's capacity for autonomous choice, to disclose information, to probe for and ensure understanding and voluntariness, and to foster adequate decision-making.

> "Temptations sometimes arise in health care for physicians and other professionals to foster or perpetuate patients' dependency, rather than to promote their autonomy. But discharging the obligation to respect patients' autonomy requires equipping them to overcome their sense of dependence and achieve as much control as possible and as they desire."[12]

This goes much further than the passive notion of informed consent which is commonly translated in practice as the need to obtain a signature from the patient or their relative to certify that information about the risks of a medical intervention has been provided and that the patient has authorized the procedure. Although ethicists have argued that informed consent implies adequate disclosure, full comprehension, voluntariness and active consent, the way in which it is implemented often seems to be designed to protect the clinician from legal liability if something goes wrong, rather than enabling the patient to make informed choices. The information provided often concerns only the procedure itself, with no discussion of alternatives. Despite the widespread acceptance by doctors of the principle of informed consent, in its practical application consent to treatment is rarely truly informed.

The question of the extent to which patients want to be actively involved in decision-making is considered in the next chapter, which will also look at ways of eliciting their role preferences, and evidence on the effects of active involvement.

Patient-centred care

The term *patient-centred care* is widely used nowadays, but there is disagreement about its origin and meaning. The ideas it embodies can be traced back over the last fifty years to the analyses of doctor-patient communication by Szasz and Hollender, Balint, and Byrne and Long.[13-15] Their calls for a new style of medical consultation were given practical expression in the 1980s by GPs such as Levenstein in South Africa and McWhinney in Canada, and by participants in the Picker/Commonwealth Program for Patient-Centred care which was established in 1987 by the Commonwealth Fund of New York.[16-18] A succinct definition of patient-centred care clearly incorporates notions of responsiveness and autonomy:

> "Patient-centred care is health care that is closely congruent with and responsive to patients' wants, needs, and preferences."[19]

Stewart proposed five domains of patient-centred care which focus specifically on the doctor's role in providing it:

Patient-centred care:
a) explores the patient's main reason for the visit, concerns, and need for information;
b) seeks an integrated understanding of the patients' world – that is, their whole person, emotional needs, and life issues;
c) finds common ground on what the problem is and mutually agrees on management;
d) enhances prevention and health promotion; and
e) enhances the continuing relationship between the patient and the doctor.[20]

This broad definition is helpful but it has proved difficult to measure the extent to which it is put into practice in everyday situations.[21] An attempt to do so by getting patients to rate their GPs in relation to various statements based on Stewart's five domains of patient-centred care produced a slightly different list of five factors: communication and partnership, personal relationship, health promotion, positive and clear approach to the problem, interest in effect on life.[22] However, it was not clear from this study whether these domains corresponded to patients' views on what they wanted, since participants were simply given questionnaires and asked to indicate the extent of their agreement with pre-selected criteria.

A different approach was adopted by the Harvard-based team leading the Picker/Commonwealth initiative.[18] They conducted qualitative research to determine patient's priorities before developing questionnaires based on what the patients in the focus groups told them were the most important factors. The aim was to measure patient's reports of the quality of care as they experienced it, rather than asking them to rate their satisfaction. These initial studies identified seven dimensions of patient-centred care as seen through the eyes of hospital inpatients:

- *Respect for patients' values, preferences, and expressed needs* (including impact of illness and treatment on quality of life, involvement in decision-making, dignity, needs and autonomy);
- *Coordination and integration of care* (including clinical care, ancillary and support services, and 'front-line' care);
- *Information, communication, and education* (including clinical status, progress and prognosis, processes of care, facilitation of autonomy, self-care and health promotion);
- *Physical comfort* (including pain management, help with activities of daily living, surroundings and hospital environment);
- *Emotional support and alleviation of fear and anxiety* (including clinical status, treatment and prognosis, impact of illness on self and family, financial impact of illness);
- *Involvement of family and friends* (including social and emotional support, involvement in decision-making, support for caregiving, impact on family dynamics and functioning);
- *Transition and continuity* (including information about medication and danger signals to look out for after leaving hospital, coordination and discharge planning, clinical, social, physical and financial support).

Changing the culture

Whatever definition of patient-centred care you espouse, it is clear that much modern health care falls considerably short of the ideal.[23-25] The changes that are needed are more than cosmetic. What is required is a change in the way clinicians and patients think about their roles, in other words a culture change. Patients' rights to make autonomous decisions need to be better understood, encouraged and supported. This is necessary to restore confidence in the system, to facilitate appropriate treatment choices, to manage care effectively, to ensure patient safety, to raise quality standards and to promote accountability. The patient needs to be seen as an active participant and the clinician as a facilitator. They should be equal partners in the process of dealing with illness. Old habits which promote dependence and passivity in patients must be cast aside, along with the paternalistic attitudes which underpin these behaviours. Clinicians will need to develop expertise in information retrieval, preference elicitation, interpretation of evidence and risk, and education for self-reliance, alongside their more traditional clinical skills.

The following chapters examine the supporting evidence for these assertions and the likely impact of greater patient and public engagement.

REFERENCES

1   Secretary of State for Health. Learning from Bristol: The report of the Public Inquiry into children's heart surgery at the Bristol Royal Infirmary 1984–95. CM5207(II). 2001. London, The Stationery Office.

2   Mercer SW, Watt GCM, Reilly D. Empathy is important for enablement (letter). British Medical Journal 2001;322:865.

3   Secretary of State for Health. The NHS Plan: a plan for investment, a plan for reform. 2000. London, Stationery Office.

4   Mulligan J. What do the public think? Health Care UK 2000;Winter:12–7.

5   Coulter, A. NICE and CHI: reducing variations and raising standards. Health Care UK 1999/2000 . 1999. London, King's Fund.

6   New B,.Rationing Agenda Group. The rationing agenda in the NHS. British Medical Journal 1996;312:1593–601.

7   Anon. Collins English Dictionary. Glasgow: Harper Collins, 1994.

8   Herxheimer A,.Goodare H. Who are you, and who are we? Looking through some key words. *Health Expectations* 1999;**2**:3–6.

9   Neuberger J. Let's do away with "patients". *British Medical Journal* 1999;**318**:1756–8.

[10] Tallis R. Commentary: leave well alone. *British Medical Journal* 1999;**318**:1757–8.

[11] Ritchie CW, Hayes D, Ames DJ. Patient or client? The opinions of people attending a psychiatric clinic. *Psychiatric Bulletin* 2000;**24**:447–50.

[12] Beauchamp TL, Childress JF. Principles of Biomedical Ethics. Oxford: Oxford University Press, 2001.

[13] Szasz TS,.Hollender MH. A contribution to the philosophy of medicine. The basic models of the doctor-patient relationship. *Archives of Internal Medicine* 1956;**97**:585–92.

[14] Balint M. The doctor, his patient and the illness. London: Pitman Medical, 1964.

[15] Byrne P, Long B. Doctors talking to patients. London: HMSO, 1976.

[16] Levenstein JH. The patient-centred general practice consultation. *South African Family Practice* 1984;**5**:276–82.

[17] McWhinney I. Patient-centred and doctor-centred models of clinical decision-making. In Sheldon M, Brook J, Roter D, eds. *Decision making in general practice*, London: Stockton, 1985.

[18] Gerteis M, Edgman-Levitan S, Daley J, Delbanco TL. Through the patient's eyes: understanding and promoting patient-centred care. San Francisco: Jossey Bass, 1993.

[19] Laine C,.Davidoff C. Patient-centred medicine: a professional evolution. *Journal of the American Medical Association* 1996;**275**:152–6.

[20] Stewart M. Toward a global definition of patient centred care. *British Medical Journal* 2001;**322**:444–5.

[21] Mead N,.Bower P. Patient-centredness: a conceptual framework and review of the empirical literature. *Social Science and Medicine* 2000;**51**:1087–110.

[22] Little P, Everitt H, Williamson I, Warner G, Moore M, Gould C *et al*. Observational study of effect of patient centredness and positive approach on outcomes of general practice consultations. *British Medical Journal* 2001;**323**:908–11.

[23] Cleary PD, Edgman-Levitan S, Roberts M, Moloney TW, McMullen W, Walker JD et al. Patients evaluate their hospital care: a national survey. *Health Affairs* 1991;**10**:254–67.

[24] Coulter A,.Cleary PD. Patients' experiences with hospital care in five countries. *Health Affairs* 2001;**20**:244–52.

[25] Lewin SA, Skea ZC, Entwistle V, Zwarenstein M, Dick J. Interventions for providers to promote a patient centred approach in clinical consultations (Cochrane Review). Oxford: Update Software, 2002.

2. Public confidence and expectations

"There is undoubtedly a growing gap between expectations and reality.
More people think that the overall state of the NHS is bad than good and
three quarters think that it has had insufficient investment. Today's
reality falls a long way short of tomorrow's vision."[1]

Wanless, D. Securing our future health: taking a long-term view.
HM Treasury, 2002

Loss of confidence

In 1999 the Commonwealth Fund organised a survey on public attitudes to
health care systems in Australia, Canada, New Zealand, UK and USA. The
survey revealed high levels of anxiety among the people most likely to need
medical care, i.e. older people on low incomes.[2] Nearly a third of low income
older people in some of these rich countries were afraid that they would be
denied access to care because they couldn't afford to pay for it. Also striking was
the level of pessimism about the quality of health care. A considerable
proportion of elderly people in most of these countries reported the impression
that standards were getting worse rather than better and a substantial number
said their health systems needed to be completely rebuilt. In Australia, Canada
and New Zealand greatest concern was expressed by people over the age of 65
while in Britain and the USA younger people were more critical of their health
systems than older people.

Why is it that so many people in the rich countries feel their health systems are in
crisis at a time when expenditures are rising and medical care is becoming more
and more effective? What has caused the loss of confidence in the NHS? Public
attitudes are influenced by knowledge of what is happening in other countries,
by what people read in newspapers or watch on television, by commercial
pressures, and by the views of health professionals. The effect of each of these on
public attitudes to health care demands closer examination.

International comparisons

Since its establishment in 1948, the NHS has been the centrepiece of the British Welfare State and its founding principle of providing needs based health care, largely free at the point of use, has continued to command widespread popular support. However, public dissatisfaction with the way in which this principle is translated into practice has been increasing. Primary care still receives high satisfaction ratings, but people have been growing more and more concerned about the quality of hospital care.[3]

A contributory factor to this loss of confidence was the sense that the NHS was no longer 'the best' health system. In the 1980s public pride in the relative efficiency and effectiveness of the NHS began to give way to a growing awareness that the service was underfunded and that health systems in other western developed countries, such as France and Germany, provided faster access and better quality care, albeit at higher cost. It became apparent that patients in the UK were being denied new technologies which were readily available elsewhere. For example, in 1980 UK per capita rates for treatment of renal failure were less than half US rates, in 1990 coronary revascularization rates were half that recommended by WHO, and prescription items per head were 47% less than in Germany, 49% less than in Spain, 62% less than in Italy and 80% less than in France.[4]

British people started to believe that the NHS was suffering the consequences of cumulative underfunding. Over the last twenty years British governments had spent considerably less on health care than most of their European counterparts, including Germany, France, the Netherlands, Austria, Switzerland, Spain, Sweden, Norway, Italy and Finland. In a comparison of health spending in 29 OECD countries only Turkey, Poland, Mexico and Korea spent a lower proportion of their gross domestic product on health care.[5] The UK's spending in 1998 was 6.8% of GDP as against the OECD average of 7.9%. In per capita terms the UK spent US $1,510 per head of population compared to Germany's $2,361 and $2,034 in France.

The NHS could, with some justification, claim to be more efficient than the health systems in many of these countries. For example, in 1992 average lengths of stay were shortest in the UK at 5.5 days compared to Germany's average of 12.6 days.[6] The relatively well organised general practice gatekeeper system was another important reason why the UK managed to hold costs down[7], but in other respects it was clear that the UK was lagging behind. Evidence was emerging that the UK had slipped down the public health league tables. Deaths from coronary heart disease were among the highest in Europe, cancer survival rates were relatively poor and the teenage pregnancy rate was particularly high.[8] In addition, many hospital buildings were in a poor state, standards in general practice and community nursing were very variable, and low pay and poor working conditions were causing recruitment difficulties, particularly among nurses and some medical specialties. There were few signs of mass exodus to the private sector, but doubt remained about the fortitude of the post-War consensus on the NHS. How much longer would people tolerate low standards of comfort, privacy and responsiveness?

The loss of confidence in health systems was not apparent everywhere. Systems in some countries retained strong public support, whereas in others there was evidence of widespread disquiet about the quality of public health care. The Eurobarometer survey carried out in 1996 in fifteen European countries revealed striking variations in the extent of dissatisfaction with health services among members of the public in the different EU Member States.[9] (Table 1)

The proportion of respondents indicating that they were fairly or very dissatisfied with the health system in their country varied from only 5% in Austria to 59% in Italy. The UK fell at the lower end of this performance scale, ranking 12th out of 15 with 41% of survey respondents indicating dissatisfaction. The results revealed a relationship between satisfaction and per capita expenditure on health. The five countries with the highest satisfaction scores (Denmark, Finland, Netherlands, Luxembourg and Belgium) spent more on health care per capita than most of those with the lowest (Greece, Portugal, Spain, Ireland and the UK). The exception was Italy which spent more than Denmark, Finland and Sweden but achieved low levels of satisfaction. In general, public support for increasing government expenditure on health care mirrored current spending rates, with more than 70% of respondents in low-spending Greece, UK, Portugal and Ireland saying the government should spend more.

Cross-national comparisons using this type of global satisfaction indicator must be treated with caution because they can produce misleading results. For example, a 1998 survey carried out by the Commonwealth Fund in Australia,

Canada, New Zealand, UK and USA asked respondents a series of factual questions about waiting times for non-emergency surgery experienced by themselves or their relatives.[10] They were also asked to comment on their level of concern about waiting times. The longest waits occurred in the UK and the shortest in the USA, with Australia, Canada and New Zealand falling between these two extremes. However, public concern about waiting times was highest in New Zealand where 38% of respondents said they were very worried. In the UK only 12% said they were very worried, the lowest proportion of all the countries. If concern about long waits was the only available measure of health system performance, it would have been easy to draw the erroneous conclusion that waiting times were not an issue in the UK.

TABLE 1

Satisfaction with health systems in the fifteen EU Member States in 1996 and per capita expenditure on health in US Purchasing Power Parities[16]

Country	% satisfied (1996)	% dissatisfied (1996)	% saying government should spend more (1996)	Per capita expenditure on health in US $ PPPs (1994)
Denmark	90.0	5.7	34.8	1362
Finland	86.4	6.0	31.8	1357
Netherlands	72.8	17.4	48.5	1641
Luxembourg	71.1	8.9	33.9	1697
Belgium	70.1	8.3	40.6	1653
Sweden	67.3	14.2	58.1	1348
Germany	66.0	10.9	25.7	1869
France	65.1	14.6	32.4	1866
Austria	63.3	4.7	16.4	1965
Ireland	59.3	29.1	71.0	1201
UK	48.1	40.9	81.5	1211
Spain	35.6	28.6	53.5	1005
Portugal	19.9	59.3	79.4	938
Greece	18.4	53.9	87.1	598
Italy	16.3	59.4	51.2	1561

Global satisfaction ratings are an imperfect measure of system performance, particularly prone to the influence of prior expectations and reporting biases. People can be satisfied with care that is not high quality and dissatisfied with high quality care. Responses may reflect the fact that outcomes were perceived to be satisfactory by respondents, even if the quality of care was not. Relief that one has survived an episode of illness may override concerns about the way care was delivered. Global satisfaction ratings may be influenced by the popularity of the government at the time of the survey, or by public confidence in economic prospects, and they are highly susceptible to media influences.[11] For example, the current media vogue for repeated headlines about long waits on trolleys in A&E departments can convince the public, and politicians, that the situation is worse than it actually is.

In 1999 54% of a random sample of British people named health as their first priority for extra government spending and 59% said the government should increase taxes and spend more.[3] Unfortunately, though, the desire for increased government spending on public services did not translate into a willingness to pay increased taxes when people were called upon to vote in general elections, with the result that NHS spending remained tightly capped throughout the 1980s and 1990s. Meanwhile rising public expectations, demographic change and the high cost of new technological developments placed the service under increased pressure until in 2002 the government finally recognised that spending would have to rise substantially.[1]

Simply spending more is unlikely to be sufficient to ensure that patients' needs are met more effectively. A health system requires appropriate incentives, checks and balances to ensure it performs well, hence the obsession with policy reform in most European countries. The Eurobarometer survey results revealed no obvious link between satisfaction rates and other aspects of health care policy, such as mode of funding (taxation or social insurance), purchaser-provider separation, price competition between providers, capitation payment for primary care doctors, controls on pharmaceutical expenditure, explicit rationing systems, or stages in the reform process. Governments in many countries have been rearranging these structural mechanisms in an attempt to achieve better value for money, but there is no clear evidence on which of these policy instruments might produce the best results from the patient's perspective.

Nevertheless, the sense that the health system is not performing optimally is not confined to the British NHS. Even high spending countries such as Germany and France have been engaged in reform programmes designed to improve value for money. What makes the British reforms different is the intense focus on improving the patient's experience. Evidence of how low public confidence in the system has fallen relative to other wealthy countries has galvanised British politicians into a desperate search for ways of increasing responsiveness to patients in the hope that this will restore confidence. The promise to raise funding levels to the European average was a direct result of this concern. However, attitudes to health care are shaped by several other influences, namely the media, healthcare industry and health professionals. Attempts to restore confidence in the NHS should take careful account of these influences as they have the power to undermine the best laid plans of politicians.

Media influences

The media is an important source of health information. Health is of prime importance to most people, so it is no surprise that the mass media reflects this interest by devoting a considerable amount of attention to stories about health risks, new treatments, patients' concerns and the politics of health care. Medical and health features are very popular and can be found in every newspaper and on most broadcasting schedules. In responding to public interest in these issues, journalists, producers and editors play an important part in shaping public expectations.

In selecting what to write about and what to publish, journalists and editors are influenced by the characteristics of the newspaper or television channel, the source of the story and the availability of specialist expertise, competition from other types of story or feature, interest from other media outlets, and their intuition and views on 'newsworthiness'. Much news is 'manufactured', in the sense that it is generated by organisations and interests external to the news media to suit a particular purpose. Journalists do not usually reproduce press releases uncritically or without looking for alternative interpretations of a particular story, but the news agenda tends to be shaped by those who have a vested interest in influencing public opinion. The views of large institutions, both statutory or public bodies and commercial corporations, tend to dominate. In the health arena these can include industrial or commercial interests, political interests, professional and patient groups.

Television drama series like *ER*, *Casualty* and *Peak Practice* provide viewers with behind-the-scenes pictures of health care which help to shape expectations of real-life health professionals and institutions. Although many such programmes strive for realism, the requirements of drama, including programme length and narrative pace, ensure that the picture they present is a distorted one.[12] Doctors and nurses are portrayed in heroic roles, patients suffer traumatic illnesses which are quickly resolved, and participants juggle stressful workloads and dramatic love-lives, apparently with impunity.

The distinction between the information and entertainment functions of the media is not as clear cut as it may at first appear. As well as informing their readers, listeners or viewers, news journalists also hope to entertain them. This can result in dramatisation of stories which begin life as dry articles in scientific journals. Reports of medical errors or unexpected adverse effects of medical treatment are often given great prominence in newspapers.[13] These have served to raise awareness of safety risks, leading to some important initiatives to tackle the problems at a system-wide level. These include exhorting health care organisations to tackle error rates by encouraging staff to speak out about the mistakes they make, and redesigning systems to make errors less likely to occur.[14] However, a media report is much more dramatic if a victim and a perpetrator can be identified and the journalistic inclination to place the blame on individuals seems set to undermine these efforts.

Evidence on the impact of media stories on health attitudes and behaviour presents a complex picture. Stories that provoke alarm can cause people to take action, sometimes with adverse consequences. For example, press coverage of research linking oral contraceptive use with an increased risk of venous thromboembolism led some women to cease taking effective contraceptives, resulting in an increase in the numbers seeking abortion.[15] Parental concern about adverse publicity surrounding childhood vaccinations for pertussis in the 1970s, and MMR nearly thirty years later, resulted in reduced immunisation rates and an increase in the incidence of serious childhood illnesses.[16] Media reports are often guilty of raising alarm about very small risks.

Stories about salmonella in eggs and chickens, BSE in cattle and genetically modified food sources have had dramatic effects on consumer behaviour, demonstrating the lengths people will go to avoid externally-imposed, and hard-to-quantify potential risks to their health. They also illustrate the increasing scepticism with which the public views reassurances from scientists and public health experts. The MMR example is classic. The more the government tries to reassure the public about the safety of the vaccine, the more sceptical the public becomes, despite the almost universal scientific consensus about the lack of connection between MMR and the risk of autism or bowel disease.[17;18] Attempts to persuade people that the risks from these health hazards are small, and indeed much smaller than those most people face with equanimity every day, such as driving a car or crossing a busy road on foot, do not seem to have the desired effect. Indeed, the lesson that bald reassuring statements by Ministers or public health experts can have the opposite effect, should have been learnt from the BSE crisis in the 1990s.[19]

The media is an important source of public information about health care and it undoubtedly shapes attitudes. Few journalists set out to deceive their readers, but they are trained to sift the dramatic story from the mundane every day reality and the effect is often to paint an overly alarming picture. The good news that most care is safe, effective and of good quality very rarely makes the front pages, but regular headlines about disasters and delays contribute to the sense that the NHS is in crisis. Small wonder that the public is growing concerned about its long-term viability.

Commercial influences

Commercial pressures can influence attitudes to, and demand for, health care. Direct-to-consumer advertising of pharmaceutical products is allowed in the USA but officially outlawed in Europe. Nevertheless the drug companies have shown themselves adept at getting publicity for their products by encouraging feature stories. The publication in 1990 of a prominent article about *Prozac* in the international news magazine Newsweek, resulted in widespread publicity in many European news media and a dramatic increase in sales of the drug.[20] Similarly, the anti-impotence drug *Viagra* became a news sensation throughout the world. Access to health information on the internet will exacerbate this trend and since the internet can be accessed from anywhere in the world, it is much harder to regulate than print media. The majority of health websites are provided or sponsored by commercial companies whose main interest is to sell their products. Indeed it is now possible to buy many drugs without prescription via the internet. For example, websites selling products such as *Viagra* (for impotence), *Zyban* (for smoking cessation), *Propecia* (for baldness) and *Meridia* (for weight loss) are relatively easy to find.[21]

Patients' requests for medicines are a powerful driver of prescribing decisions and pharmaceutical companies are well aware of this. A recent report by the Consumers' Association charted the development of direct-to-consumer advertising in the US, from the mid 1980s when the first 'disease awareness' advertisements (which didn't mention specific products) appeared in print and on TV, through the early 1990s when print advertisements for specific drugs began to appear, to 1997 when television advertisements for prescription-only products were allowed, with interactive websites providing back-up information.[22] According to this report, US spending on drugs rose by $42.7 billion in the five years from 1993 to 1998 and 22 per cent of this increase was accounted for by the ten most heavily advertised drugs.

Pharmaceutical companies have teamed up with health professionals and patient groups to raise awareness of under-diagnosed and under-treated problems. These disease awareness campaigns are legal in Europe as long as they don't mention specific products, but this practice has been dubbed 'disease mongering' because of its effect in raising concerns among basically healthy people.[23] Industry spokespersons argue that they are simply meeting the public demand for more information about health and health care, but this is disingenuous. They are adept at getting around advertising restrictions to promote their products. Advertising clearly works. Studies in the USA have shown that patients are much more likely to request and be prescribed advertised products.[24] There are concerns that recent moves by the European Commission to allow pharmaceutical companies to provide information for patients on company websites will add to the pressure for increased prescribing of possibly inappropriate treatments.[25] Commercial promotion of diseases or treatments can encourage perfectly healthy people to think they need medical attention.[26] This increases the likelihood that demand will be distorted and resources will be diverted away from those who really need them. Continuing regulation of industry's promotional efforts is essential to counter these distorting effects and to ensure equitable distribution of the public resources spent on health care.

Medical influences

Health professionals, particularly GPs, are frequently cited as the most important source of information about health and illness. A recent population survey ranked them top of the list of information sources, followed by pharmacists, family and friends, other health professionals and telephone helplines.[27] This is not at all surprising, but it underscores the importance of the doctor's role in shaping expectations. Their response to patients' requests and the way in which they define and manage health problems has considerable power to reinforce or change attitudes to healthcare.

The reliance on doctors to define and articulate health needs is an important reason why the patient role is different from that of a consumer in the commercial marketplace. When buying a car, we may understand very little about how the engine functions, but it is not too difficult to make an independent assessment of our transport needs and to choose a car which has the characteristics that we've identified as important. In health care, on the other hand, we rely on health professionals to assess our needs and to decide whether or not we have a problem which requires their intervention. In this sense the doctor is the patient's agent. However, if the agent is also the supplier of services, the separation of demand from supply – one of the essential characteristics of a properly functioning market – no longer holds. The relationship depends on the patient's trust in the doctor and in the various regulatory systems. If trust proves insufficient to guarantee high quality care, it must be supplemented with additional safeguards, hence the resort to external regulation and performance monitoring, now a universal trend.

Expectations of health care are subjective and relative. They arise from personal experience, from the political and cultural context, from knowledge of what is possible and from comparisons with other sectors or other countries. They are shaped by a variety of influences including the attitudes and beliefs of healthcare providers, especially doctors. Tudor Hart has argued that popular faith in the NHS was sustained for the first forty years of its existence by deliberately limiting expectations to what the NHS could afford within the resources allowed by government.[4] This task was tacitly accepted by most doctors and its message agreed by most patients:

> "Reasons for this essentially voluntary restraint were complex, including traditional condescension by doctors and deference to them, respect by both doctors and patients for a service based on gift relationships and trust, scepticism, stoicism, and denial of illness............NHS doctors persuaded themselves and their patients that sceptical approaches to new and costly techniques were in patients' personal interests, and were not

just ways to save money. Such claims by government would not have
been believed, but when endorsed by doctors, patients by and large
accepted their judgement."[4]

This consensus on the need for restraint could only be sustained while British
people and their doctors remained ignorant of trends elsewhere. It began to
collapse when news filtered through that the British health system was achieving
worse results than those in other countries. One of the effects of globalisation is
the rapid spread of ideas. British conservatism about medical intervention was
in sharp contrast to the view that prevailed in the USA. Americans were much
less concerned about equitable provision and much more inclined to believe that
high rates of medical intervention were an unalloyed good thing, at least for
those who could afford them. This view was fuelled by the commercial culture of
American medicine and the fee-for-service payment system, whereby doctors
had a direct pecuniary interest in encouraging demand for their services. High
intervention rates were further encouraged by high rates of litigation, which
fostered defensive practice. The result was an aggressive medical culture in
which errors of omission seemed worse than errors of commission.[4]

These ideas began to spread across the Atlantic affecting public and professional
expectations of what should be provided. Meanwhile there was growing
concern in the USA that the rate of increase in healthcare costs was causing
damage to the economy. There were calls to modify incentives by managing the
health care market and restricting the power of the main suppliers, i.e. the
doctors. The result was a shift to prospective payment schemes or 'managed
care' and an increased emphasis on external regulation.

The shift to managed care in the USA and the adoption of more market-based
systems in much of Europe signified a growing convergence of approaches to
health policy. This was accompanied by a convergence of attitudes at the
professional level. British doctors did not face the same economic incentives as
American ones, but they read the same journals, in many cases attended the
same conferences, and they were well aware of the potential benefits of new
technologies available elsewhere but denied to their patients because of
underfunding in the NHS. Many were also aware of the complaints of
American doctors about growing managerial control and they felt themselves

subject to the same constraints.[28] In addition, they felt overworked and
undersupported. In the BMA's national survey of GP opinion published in
October 2001 66% of respondents said their morale was very or fairly low, and
65% said it was worse than it had been five years previously.[29] Just as British
doctors had influenced patients' expectations about what could reasonably be
expected from the NHS in its early years, so their growing disillusion with the
system was communicated to their patients.

The BMJ's editor, Richard Smith, has suggested there may be even more
fundamental reasons why doctors appear to be increasingly unhappy.[30] In
addition to the uncomfortable sense that their role is changing in unpredictable
ways and their autonomy is being undermined, doctors' growing awareness of
the disjunction between over-optimistic ideas about the benefits of medical care
and the limitations on what they can in reality do for patients has placed them in
a difficult position (see Box 1).

Box 1

Doctors and patients: the bogus contract [30]

The patient's view
- Modern medicine can do remarkable things: it can solve many of my problems
- You, the doctor, can see inside me and know what's wrong
- You know everything it's necessary to know
- You can solve my problems, even my social problems
- So we give you high status and a good salary

The doctor's view
- Modern medicine has limited powers
- Worse, it's dangerous
- We can't begin to solve all problems, especially social ones
- I don't know everything, but I do know how difficult many things are
- The balance between doing good and harm is very fine
- I'd better keep quiet about all this so as not to disappoint my patients and lose my status.

Smith saw the problem as lying in the psychology of doctor-patient interactions,
but in a subsequent BMJ article Ham and Alberti sketched out a broader,

sociological explanation of why both doctors and patients had lost confidence in the system.[31] In their view rising expectations had been fuelled by increasing affluence and a widening gap between people's experiences in other sectors of consumption and public services. People were becoming better informed, more demanding, less deferential, more vociferous, more aware of the likelihood that things could go wrong and more willing to resort to legal action if they did. Medical self-regulation had come under fire and the government had begun to usurp the power of health professionals by encouraging external regulation. Whether you favour the psychological or the sociological explanation, the net effect has been to increase doctors' sense of frustration which they in turn have communicated to their patients.

Encouraging false expectations

Exaggerated ideas about the benefits of medical interventions are partly the result of the spread of American ideas referred to above, partly due to commercial pressures and media influences, and partly a result of the paternalistic nature of healthcare delivery in the NHS. Instead of providing patients with new knowledge, self-help and coping skills, the effect of many medical consultations is to encourage them to rely on health professionals to solve their problems, even when this is unrealistic.

A classic example is the management of low back pain. This is one of the most common health problems: 70–85% of the population will experience it at some time in their lives.[32] It is one of the most common reasons for taking sick leave from work and hence has an important impact on economic performance. Estimates suggest musculoskeletal problems are responsible for around 25 million lost working days at a cost to the economy of more than 4 billion pounds in any one year.[33] It is undoubtedly an important and distressing problem, but it is usually self-limiting: almost 90% of patients with acute low back pain get better quite rapidly, regardless of therapy. The remaining 10% are at risk of developing chronic pain and disability, and account for the majority of the social costs of back pain.[34]

Lay people have many misconceptions about the causes of this very common problem and how it can be effectively managed. The popular view that it is usually due to a slipped disk or trapped nerve is widespread, despite the fact that these probably account for less than 5% of all episodes of back pain.[35] Large numbers of back pain sufferers consult their doctors in a fruitless search for a cure, only to be referred on for more consultations with other health professionals who have little to offer.[36] Many are referred for X-ray examination. Radiography of the lumbar spine accounts for 5% of all radiographic examinations in NHS hospitals, yet there is no evidence of benefit from these investigations.[37] More than 50 different therapies are on offer, but there is sound evidence of efficacy for very few of them.[38]

The most effective strategies in the management of chronic low back pain involve maintenance of activity and behavioural therapy which teaches patients relaxation techniques and how to control the intensity of their pain.[39] Honest information, reassurance and education about strategies for self-help and prevention are probably the best way to treat this condition in its acute phase. Yet, despite this evidence, many sufferers are still encouraged to adopt a passive approach, with X-ray, bed rest and analgesics the most frequently prescribed interventions, and studies suggest that GPs are doing little to educate their patients or challenge their misconceptions.[35] If doctors are unable or unwilling to tell their patients when medical care can do little to help, it is hardly surprising that patients keep coming back searching for explanations and cures. This leads to frustration among doctors and dissatisfaction among patients.[40]

Doctors and their patients must be persuaded to acknowledge the limits of medical care. There is not, and never will be, a pill for every ill and encouraging false hopes does no one any good. Evidence-based medicine teaches health professionals to look more critically at the therapies they are trained to provide and in many cases the new knowledge provides an important challenge to traditional clinical practice. But the skills in critical appraisal that most trainee doctors now learn need to be transmitted to their patients. If doctors are encouraged to rethink traditional approaches but patients are left in ignorance, the result will be conflict and dissatisfaction.

Tackling this problem is by no means easy, because the culture of medical care encourages a 'can do' approach and this is what patients seem to want also.[41] Various attempts to provide one-off educational interventions for patients with back pain have had only limited success. A randomised controlled trial of an educational booklet for patients consulting their GPs about back pain resulted in a small reduction in referrals and in subsequent consultations for back pain.[42]

Another study found that a booklet together with a 15-minute session with a nurse improved patients' knowledge and satisfaction in an American managed care setting.[40]

Empathy and reassurance may be even more important when scientific medicine has little to offer.[43] The failure to provide this leaves the patient without support to deal with their pain, resulting in frustration and more desperate help-seeking. Public education can lead to improvements in the understanding of the condition among patients and their GPs, and this in turn can reduce both the disability caused by back pain and the costs.[44] Doctors should ensure that their patients are supplied with honest information if medicine has nothing to offer. There is no merit in perpetuating false hopes.

Future trends
Public expectations are changing and clinical practice and the organisation of health care delivery must change too if the consensual basis for publicly-funded health care systems is to survive. Greater public awareness of quality failures and medical errors will fuel the demand for external scrutiny and public accountability of health systems. International comparisons will drive up expectations among British patients, possibly weakening support for the NHS. Media and commercial influences, including disease awareness campaigns, will foster demand for wider availability of expensive treatments, including 'lifestyle' drugs and alternative therapies. The trend towards medicalisation of normal life processes, such as childbirth, psychological wellbeing, sexuality and ageing, will continue encouraged by professional and commercial interests.[45-48] Patients will need help to enable them to become more discriminating consumers of health care and doctors will need help if they are to facilitate this process.

It is too easy to blame patients for unrealistic expectations or politicians for encouraging these. Clinicians carry a share of the responsibility for loss of confidence in the NHS and they are an important part of the solution. The patient of the future will be better informed, less deferential, and less willing to tolerate poor quality care. They will expect more involvement and more choice when it comes to their own care and that of their family. Meeting these needs will place considerable pressures on the NHS. Ignoring them may make the current system unsustainable.

REFERENCES

[1]   Wanless, D. Securing our future health: taking a long-term view (final report). 2002. London, HM Treasury.

[2]   Donelan K, Blendon RJ, Schoen S, Binns K, Osborn R, Davis K. The elderly in five nations: the importance of universal coverage. *Health Affairs* 2000;19:226–35.

[3]   Mulligan J. What do the public think? *Health Care* UK 2000;**Winter**:12–7.

[4]   Tudor Hart J. Expectations of health care: promoted, managed or shared? *Health Expectations* 1998;1:1–2.

[5]   OECD. Health Data 98: A comparative analysis of twenty-nine countries. 2001. Paris, Organization for Economic Cooperation and Development.

[6]   Rosleff, F. and Lister, G. European healthcare trends: towards managed care in Europe. 1995. London, Coopers and Lybrand.

[7]   Starfield B. Is primary care essential? *Lancet* 1994;344:1129–33.

[8]   Wanless, D. Securing our future: taking a long-term view. 2001. London, HM Treasury.

[9]   Mossialos, E. Citizens and health systems: main results from Eurobarometer survey. 1998. European Commission, Directorate General for Employment, Industrial Relations and Social Affairs.

[10] Donelan K, Blendon RJ, Schoen C, Davis K, Binns K. The cost of health system change: public discontent in five nations. *Health Affairs* 1999;18:206–16.

[11] Judge K,.Solomon M. Public opinion and the National Health Service: patterns and perspectives in consumer satisfaction. *Journal of Social Policy* 1993;**22**:299–327.

[12] Turow J. Television entertainment and the US health-care debate. *Lancet* 2001;**347**:1240–3.

[13] Berwick DM. Not again! *British Medical Journal* 2001;**322**:247–8.

[14] Department of Health. An organisation with a memory: report of an expert group on learning from adverse events in the NHS. 2000. London, Stationery Office.

[15] Drife JO. The third generation pill controversy ("continued"). *British Medical Journal* 2001;**323**:119–20.

[16] Nicoll A, Elliman D, Ross E. MMR vaccination and autism 1998: Deja-vu pertussis and brain damage 1974? *British Medical Journal* 1998;**316**:715–6.

[17] Taylor B, Miller E, Lingam R, Andrews N, Simmons A, Stowe J. Measles, mumps, and rubella vaccination and bowel problems or developmental regression in children with autism: population study. *British Medical Journal* 2002;**324**:393–6.

[18] Kmietowicz Z. Government launches intensive media campaign on MMR. *British Medical Journal* 2002;**324**:383.

[19] Klein R. The politics of risk: the case of BSE. *British Medical Journal* 2000;**321**:1091–2.

[20] Nelkin D. An uneasy relationship: the tensions between medicine and the media. *Lancet* 1996;**347**:1600–3.

[21] Medications. www.pill-shop.com 2002.

[22] Consumers Association. Promotion of prescription drugs: public health or private profit? 2001. London, Consumers Association.

23 Moynihan R, Heath I, Henry D. Selling sickness: the pharmaceutical industry and disease mongering. *British Medical Journal* 2002;324:886–91.

24 Mintzes B, Barer ML, Kravitz RL, Kazanjian A, Bassett K, Lexchin J et al. Influence of direct to consumer pharmaceutical advertising and patients' requests on prescribing decisions: two site cross sectional survey. *British Medical Journal* 2002;324:278–9.

25 Medawar, C. Health, pharma and the EU: direct-to-consumer drug promotion. 2002. London, Social Audit.

26 Mintzes B. Direct to consumer advertising is medicalising normal human experience. *British Medical Journal* 2002;324:908–11.

27 Wyatt JC. Information for patients. *Journal of the Royal Society of Medicine* 2001;**93**:467–71.

28 Blendon RJ, Schoen C, Donelan K, Osborn R, DesRoches CM, Scoles K *et al.* Physicians' views on quality of care: a five-country comparison. *Health Affairs* 2001;**20**:233–43.

29 BMA. Physicians' survey highlights low morale. www.bma.org.uk . 2002.

30 Smith R. Why are doctors so unhappy? *British Medical Journal* 2001;**322**:1073–4.

31 Ham C,.Alberti KGMM. The medical profession, the public, and the government. *British Medical Journal* 2002;**324**:838–42.

32 Andersson GBJ. Epidemiological features of chronic low back pain. *Lancet* 1999;**354**:581–5.

33 Health and Safety Executive. Revitalising health and safety. 1999. London, Health and Safety Executive.

34 Waddell G. The back pain revolution. London: Churchill Livingstone, 1998.

35 Klaber Moffett JA, Newbronner E, Waddell G, Croucher K, Spear S. Public perceptions about low back pain and its management: a gap between expectations and reality? *Health Expectations* 2000;**3**:161–8.

36 Coulter A, Bradlow J, Martin-Bates C, Agass M, Tulloch A. Outcome of general practitioner referrals to specialist outpatient clinics for back pain. *British Journal of General Practice* 1991;**41**:450–3.

37 Kendrick D, Fielding K, Bentley E, Kerslake R, Miller P, Pringle M. Radiography of the lumbar spine in primary care patients with low back pain: randomised controlled trial. *British Medical Journal* 2001;**322**:400–5.

38 Van Tulder MW, Koes BW, Bouter LM. Conservative treatment of acute and chronic non-specific low back pain: a systematic review of randomised controlled trials of the most common interventions. *Spine* 1997;**22**:2128–56.

39 Van Tulder MW, Ostelo RWJG, Vlaeyen JWS, Linton SJ, Morley SJ, Assendelft WJJ. Behavioural treatment for chronic low back pain (Cochrane Review). *The Cochrane Library*, Oxford: Update Software, 2000.

40 Cherkin DC, Deyo RA, Street JH, Hunt M, Barlow W. Limited success of a program for back pain in primary care. *Spine* 1996;**21**:345–55.

41 Thomas KB. General practice consultations: is there any point in being positive? *British Medical Journal* 1987;**294**:1200–2.

[42] Roland M,.Dixon M. Randomized controlled trial of an educational booklet for patients presenting with back pain in general practice. *Journal of the Royal College of General Practitioners* 1989;**39**:244–6.

[43] Hadler N. Point of view. *Spine* 1996;**21**:355.

[44] Buchbinder R, Jolley D, Wyatt M. Population based intervention to change back pain beliefs and disability: three part evaluation. *British Medical Journal* 2001;**322**:1516–20.

[45] Johanson R, Newburn M, Macfarlane A. Has the medicalisation of childbirth gone too far? *British Medical Journal* 2002;**324**:892–5.

[46] Double D. The limits of psychiatry. *British Medical Journal* 2002;**324**:900–4.

[47] Hart G,.Wellings K. Sexual behaviour and its medicalisation: in sickness and in health. *British Medical Journal* 2002;**324**:896–900.

[48] Ebrahim S. The medicalisation of old age. *British Medical Journal* 2002;**324**:816–63.

3. Choosing appropriate treatment: patient as decision-maker

"If communication is to a degree possible between experts in some areas
of the modern world why not between doctors (with one sort of
expertise) and patients (with another)?"[1]

Tuckett,D. et al. Meetings between experts. Tavistock, 1985

Do patients want to participate in treatment decisions?

It used to be assumed that doctors and patients shared the same goals and that
only the doctor was sufficiently informed and experienced to decide what should
be done. Patients are now much more likely to challenge the notion that 'doctor
knows best'. A hundred years ago doctors expected patients to follow their
advice without question. Patients' views and preferences were seen as irrelevant
and requests for additional information were often dismissed. In 1871 Oliver
Wendell Holmes gave the following advice to American medical students:

"Your patient has no more right to all the truth you know than he has to
all the medicine in your saddlebags. He should get only just so much as is
good for him."[2]

Nowadays failures in communication of information about illness and
treatment are the most frequent source of patient dissatisfaction.[3,4] There is
plenty of evidence that most patients want more information than they are
currently given, but this does not necessarily mean they want to participate in
decision-making. Some clinicians have argued that the desire for greater
involvement is restricted to a minority group of young, white, middle class
patients, but the evidence does not support this. These groups are often better
able to articulate their preferences, but attitudes are changing fast and age or
social class is by no means a reliable guide to what patients want.

A number of studies have investigated the extent of desire for participation
among different groups of patients. For example, in a study of 439 interactions
between adult cancer patients and oncologists in an American hospital, the

majority (92%) preferred to be given all information including bad news, and two thirds (69%) said they wanted to participate in treatment decisions.[5] Meanwhile, somewhat different results were produced by a Canadian study which looked at information and participation preferences among 52 outpatients undergoing post-surgical treatment for cancer.[6] Almost two-thirds (63%) felt the doctor should take the primary responsibility in decision-making, 27% felt it should be an equally shared process, and 10% felt they should take the major role.

Certain patients, especially older ones, may prefer a paternalistic consulting style. For example, a study by a British GP found that his patients were more satisfied when he adopted a 'directing' style than when he emphasised 'sharing', although the author didn't reveal what his 'normal' style was, nor how skilled he was in offering the two types of consultation.[7] An abrupt switch of style could be confusing to patients used to something different. Even if some people are more comfortable with the old-fashioned approach, there are signs of increasing frustration with paternalistic attitudes and failure to take account of patients' views and preferences. In a survey of 2,249 patients recently discharged from hospital in the UK, 20% said staff didn't always treat them with respect and dignity, 29% said that doctors sometimes talked about them in front of them as if they weren't there, and 59% said they were not given enough say in treatment decisions.[8]

Desire for participation has been found to vary according to age, educational status, disease severity and cultural background. A study of 256 American cancer patients found that younger patients were more likely to want active participation in decisions about their care, but a substantial proportion of older patients also wanted to be involved: 87% of patients aged under 40 expressed a desire to participate, compared to 62% of those aged 40–59 and 51% of those aged over 60.[9] Some people prefer to leave the final decision about treatment options to the doctor, but they may still want to be involved in the decision-making process. A study of a group of older patients with coronary heart disease revealed considerable dissatisfaction about the fact that they were given very little encouragement or opportunity to participate in decisions about their care and little attempt had been made to inform them about the treatment options.[10] They felt this implied a lack of respect for their views on the part of the doctors.

An age-related trend has been found in a number of studies – younger and better educated people are more likely to want to play an active role.[5;11-17] This raises the interesting question of whether this is simply an age effect or whether it is a cohort effect. In other words, is it the case that older people are naturally more passive than younger people, or does it indicate that the preference for active involvement is increasing over time, suggestive of a cultural change? Cross-sectional studies such as these cannot provide a definitive answer, but it seems very likely that the latter is true, perhaps reflecting greater knowledge of the potential harms as well as the benefits of medical care and decreased willingness to submit to the authority of clinicians. Views are likely to change as patients experience effective examples of participation.

Despite the association between age and decision-making preferences, age on its own is not a reliable predictor of a patient's preferred role. Older people are particularly likely to suffer from the presumption that they are incapable of taking decisions or unwilling to face choices about their medical care. Care of patients at the end of life is a case in point. National guidance requires that do-not-rescuscitate orders should not be applied without first discussing the issue with patients and/or their relatives, yet there is evidence that this does not happen in two-thirds of cases.[18] Respect for autonomy is just as important at the end of life as at any other time and arguments that the patient cannot comprehend the choices they face are not defensible as a reason for avoiding the attempt to involve them.[19]

People's preferences may vary according to the stage in the course of a disease episode and the severity of their condition. Another Canadian study found a much greater desire for active participation among a randomly selected population sample than among a group of newly diagnosed cancer patients, pointing to the difficulty in predicting the level of involvement desired when serious illness strikes.[20] There may also be important cultural differences. Studies comparing responses in different countries found that British breast cancer patients were less likely to prefer an active role than Canadian ones.[21,22] However trials in the UK of interventions designed to inform patients and enable them to play a more active role have been well received by people in all social groups.[23-25]

Although many patients want to participate in decision-making, it is important to remember that it is also legitimate to choose a more passive role. Schneider has criticised the tendency to assume that autonomy is mandatory, in other words that patients must make decisions personally whenever feasible.[26] Some patients may not want to exercise their autonomy and this should be respected. A requirement to make choices could place an additional and unwanted burden on people who are sick, possibly with harmful results.

Clearly it is not desirable to force people to make choices if they don't want to, but the difficulty facing the clinician is to know what role an individual patient wants to play in a particular circumstance and how to facilitate this in a sensitive manner. The assumption that sick people do not want to participate in decisions about their care, if unchecked, takes us right back to square one, i.e. paternalism and the denial of autonomy. It is important, therefore, to explore patients' role preferences and to offer full information and involvement wherever significant choices must be made.[27] The wishes of the patient who chooses not to make a choice must be respected, but the option of involvement should be offered wherever practical.

Different styles of decision-making

Most patients expect to be given information about their condition and the treatment options and they want clinicians to take account of their preferences. This points to the need for new styles of decision-making in clinical practice. Decision theorists differ over the number of models of clinical decision-making they distinguish and the terminology they use to describe them, but there is broad agreement that there are at least three distinctly different approaches (see Box 1).[28-30]

Box 1

Models of clinical decision-making		
Professional choice	*Shared decision-making*	*Consumer choice*
Clinician decides, patient consents	Information shared, both decide together	Clinician informs, patient makes decision

The traditional model – I have termed it the *professional choice* model – assumed that doctors and patients shared the same goals, that only the doctor was sufficiently informed and experienced to decide what should be done, and patient involvement was limited to giving or withholding consent to treatment. The *consumer choice* model assumes that the patient alone will make the decision once he/she has been provided with all necessary technical information. The patient's preferences are pre-eminent in this model and the clinician's role is reduced to that of information provider.

In *shared decision-making*, on the other hand, the intention is that both the process of decision-making and the outcome – the treatment decision – will be shared. This is a partnership approach based on the notion that two types of expertise are involved. The doctor is, or should be, well informed about diagnostic techniques, the causes of disease, prognosis, treatment options, and preventive strategies, but only the patient knows about his or her experience of illness, social circumstances, habits and behaviour, attitudes to risk, values and preferences. Both types of knowledge are needed to manage illness successfully, so both parties should be prepared to share information and take decisions jointly. Shared information is an essential prerequisite, but the process also depends on a commitment from both parties to engage in a negotiated decision-making process. The clinician must provide the patient with information about diagnosis, prognosis and treatment options, including outcome probabilities, and the patient must be prepared to discuss their values and preferences. The clinician must acknowledge the legitimacy of the patient's preferences and the patient has to accept shared responsibility for the treatment decision.

While paternalism seems largely inappropriate in modern medical care, it would be wrong to assume that there is no place for professional choice. Each of these modes of decision-making has its place in particular clinical settings – the trick is to match the appropriate style to the patient's needs at any particular time. For example, emergency situations often require clinicians to make quick decisions when there is no time to involve the patient, or the patient may be comatose or incapable of active participation for some reason. In these cases the professional choice model is entirely appropriate. In other situations it may be appropriate to leave the final decision to the patient, with the clinician's role relegated to provider of technical information as implied in the consumer choice model. Examples might include a woman's choice of contraceptive method – assuming she has full information about efficacy and risks and there are no relevant contra-indications, the woman who wants to should be allowed to decide for herself. The clinician has to use his/her knowledge of the individual patient to determine the most appropriate style of decision-making. In most cases the choice for the clinician will fall between eliciting the patient's preferences and using this information to make a decision about the most appropriate treatment if the patient prefers to rely on the doctor's recommendation, or actively involving the patient in making the decision.

Consent or choice?

While informed consent is a legal requirement for surgical procedures and for entry into clinical trials, it is not mandatory for other medical interventions. Nevertheless, the UK General Medical Council (GMC) considers that obtaining informed consent to diagnostic and screening procedures and all treatments is part of a doctor's ethical obligations. To facilitate this the GMC considers it essential that doctors provide patients with sufficient information to make a fully informed choice.[31] Successive British Governments have made statements in support of this view. In 1992 the Patient's Charter informed British patients that they have the right "*to be given a clear explanation of any treatment proposed, including any risks and any alternatives, before you decide whether you will agree to the treatment.*"[32] And the NHS Plan, published in 2000, promised patients much greater information about their treatment.[33] Yet it is still the case that many patients say they are not given full information about their treatments or a real opportunity to have a say in decisions about their care.[34]

The problem is that informed consent has been viewed as an essentially passive activity, at least as far as patients undergoing treatment are concerned. The way doctors refer to it illustrates the point. They tend to talk about "consenting the patient", using it as a transitive verb as if consent were something that's done to the patient like being given an injection, rather than an active decision by the patient. Frequently a junior doctor is despatched to get the patient's consent, the trophy being the required signature on the consent form. Often this occurs long after the decision about treatment has actually been taken, for example while the patient is being prepared for surgery. The doctor may offer information about the operation, but at this stage the patient may not be in a frame of mind to take it in. One study found that 60% of surgical patients were poorly informed about the procedure they were about to undergo immediately after admission to hospital, yet 69% signed the consent form without reading it.[35] The device of the consent form and the pre-surgical information session is primarily to protect doctors against litigation.[36] The patient's failure to absorb the information or to read the form is unsurprising if it is presented at a time when acquiescence to treatment is virtually irrevocable.

What do patients need to make informed choices?

The General Medical Council (GMC) tells doctors:

> "It is for the patient, not the doctor, to determine what is in the patient's own best interests. You may wish to recommend a treatment or a course of action, but you must not put pressure on patients to accept your advice."[31]

They insist that doctors should provide full information to enable the patient to make a choice. They should elicit patients' views and preferences, answer their questions honestly, use written material and visual aids where appropriate, and allow sufficient time for patients to absorb the information and discuss it with others if they wish. For this to be feasible, doctors need training in how to impart information about risk and probability and how to answer patients' questions. Some questions commonly asked by patients are summarised in Box 2:

Box 2

Patients' Questions

Diagnosis:
- What is wrong with me?
- What is causing the problem?
- How does my experience compare with that of others with the same problem?
- What are the tests for?
- How certain is the diagnosis?

Treatment:
- What are the treatment options?
- What are the potential benefits and harms of each of these?
- Will treatment relieve the symptoms?
- Is treatment essential?
- How long will it take to recover?
- What effect will it have on my quality of life?

Screening:
- What is the purpose of screening?
- How accurate is the test?

continued

- What is the probability of a false positive or false negative result?
- Are there any other likely benefits or harms?
- Will further investigation be necessary?
- If a disease is detected, how effective is the subsequent treatment?
- Will I have access to counselling or support if necessary?

Many clinicians are attracted to the idea of a participative decision-making style in theory, but find it difficult to put into practice. Time constraints inhibit information provision and it is sometimes quite difficult to discover what the patient already knows and how much they want to be involved. Shared decision-making involves sharing information about the limitations and risks of treatment as well as the benefits. Some clinicians fear that encouraging patients to choose between competing treatment options will place an additional burden on people who are feeling unwell, causing unnecessary anxiety and distress.[37] Some patients may prefer an optimistic rather than a realistic account of their chances of recovery.

A Canadian study of patients with early stage breast cancer found that patients' desire to adopt a positive approach to fighting their illness resulted in a tendency to want more aggressive interventions, notwithstanding the risks of the treatment.[38] For example, patients tended to overestimate the possible benefits of chemotherapy and downplay the risks. If a more evidence-based approach to treatment decision-making is to be encouraged, it will be important to avoid undermining patients' coping strategies by invalidating their values and beliefs. Active involvement implies accepting responsibility for the outcomes of treatment even when these are adverse.

Patients with life-threatening illnesses, such as cancer, may be less willing to accept shared responsibility than those with less serious conditions. In these cases it may be more important to allow patients an opportunity to express their concerns and preferences than to involve them in the decision itself. Studies in which breast cancer patients were offered a choice between mastectomy or breast-conserving surgery found no ill-effects of involving patients in the decision, but the findings conflicted on whether offering choice led to psychological benefits.[39-41] Decision-making in cases of serious illness can be a protracted process. Patients require time to come to terms with the choices facing them and seek a sympathetic hearing from the clinician.

Patients require information for a variety of purposes. A qualitative study of patients' information needs, involving focus groups of patients with a variety of common conditions, identified a number of reasons why they needed information, including the following:

- to understand what is wrong
- to gain a realistic idea of prognosis
- to make the most of consultations
- to understand the processes and likely outcomes of tests and treatments
- to assist in self-care
- to learn about available services and sources of help
- to provide reassurance and help to cope
- to help others (family, friends, carers, employers, etc.) understand what they're going through
- to legitimise help-seeking and concerns
- to identify further information and sources of support
- to identify the 'best' health care providers.[42]

All these items of information are necessary if patients are to become active participants in their care. Some questions may be hard to answer because the information is uncertain or unavailable or not provided in a format that matches what patients want to know.[43] An evidence-based approach is as important for patients as it is for clinicians, but lack of evidence does not justify the omission of information about common treatments or possible outcomes. In the real world of clinical practice decisions often have to be made on the basis of incomplete evidence and it is important that patients understand the inherent uncertainties. Patients' information needs may change during the course of an illness. For example, at the time of first onset or diagnosis it may be more relevant to provide details of the tests and investigations used and descriptive information about the condition and prognosis. Depending on the condition, it may be appropriate to provide detailed information about specific treatments at a later stage.

How can patients' access to information be improved?

As we have seen, evidence exists that many patients have strong treatment preferences, that these are not always predictable, and that doctors often fail to understand them. Patients cannot express informed preferences unless they are given sufficient and appropriate information, including detailed explanations about their condition and the likely outcomes with and without treatment.

Consultation times are limited – there is often insufficient time to explain fully the condition and the treatment choices. Health professionals may themselves lack knowledge of treatment options and their effects. Patients find it hard to know what questions to ask.

A solution to this problem is to ensure that patients have access to good quality written or audiovisual material, to inform themselves and to use in discussion with health professionals. A recent survey of patient information materials currently in use in the NHS found that the quality of most materials was poor: many leaflets or audio-visual aids contained inaccurate and out-of-date information; topics that patients considered important were omitted; much information was biased, giving a one-sided and often optimistic view of the benefits of medical interventions, risks and side-effects were inadequately described, controversies and uncertainties were glossed over, and information about treatment effectiveness was often missing or unreliable.[34]

If decision-making is to be shared, the information to inform decisions must also be shared. Patients must be given help to obtain the information they need. Given the short consultation times experienced in most busy clinics, it is often unrealistic to expect clinicians to provide full information about the risks and benefits of all treatment options. This information is not always readily available to clinicians, let alone lay people. If patients are to be able to express their preferences, they require help in the form of user-friendly information packages or decision aids.

Research into the use of decision aids for patients has shown that they can be an effective solution to these problems. When patient participation is facilitated by using specially designed decision aids, their knowledge and satisfaction with the decision process is increased.[44;45] In a recent study 205 women facing a decision about whether or not to take hormone replacement therapy (HRT) were randomly allocated to one of two groups.[23] The intervention group saw an interactive video which summarised the evidence on the benefits and harms of this treatment, including the effect on menopausal symptoms and on health and well being in the longer term. The control group received 'normal care'. Of the women randomised to the video 82% said they found it very easy to understand and 85% said it increased their knowledge of HRT. Decisional conflict (the extent to which people feel comfortable with their decisions) was significantly lower (better) in the intervention group than in the control group and the video was successful in helping women to make up their mind about the most appropriate action for them. A similar study of a decision aid for patients with benign prostatic hypertrophy demonstrated that these information packages were also found acceptable and useful by a relatively elderly group of men.[24]

Decision aids help people make specific deliberative decisions about disease management and treatment options, prevention or screening. They use a variety of media to present the information in an accessible form to patients, including leaflets, audiotapes, workbooks, decision boards, computer programmes, interactive videos, web sites, structured interviews, and group presentations. The content is based on reviews of clinical research and studies of patients' information needs. They are very different from standard health education materials because they are not didactic or prescriptive – they do not tell people what to do. Instead they help patients clarify their own values and preferences and weigh up the potential benefits and harms of alternative courses of action.

Decision aids have been developed to cover a variety of types of medical decision; for example, conditions where there is more than one possible treatment option (e.g. benign prostatic hypertrophy (BPH), back pain, breast cancer, menstrual problems, etc.); interventions where patient's choice is paramount (e.g. circumcision, contraception, etc.); diagnostic tests or screening programmes (e.g. amniocentesis, PSA, mammography); preventive therapies or behaviours (e.g. HRT, vaccinations, risk factors for coronary heart disease, etc.); the management of chronic diseases (e.g. arthritis, diabetes, asthma, etc.); and end-of-life decisions (e.g. resuscitation). Decision aids are not required in every situation. They are not necessary when there is strong evidence in favour of a specific intervention and there are no appropriate alternatives, in emergency situations, or when a patient has made it clear that they do not want to participate in decisions about their care.

Good decision aids include evidence-based statements of benefits and risks derived from credible sources, refer to the quality and consistency of empirical studies and are explicit about uncertainties and controversies, present all options (including doing nothing) in a balanced way, and are well designed, clearly structured and concise.[46] Many decision aids use interactive methods to help patients clarify their values. It is important that they are kept up-to-date and revised when new evidence emerges, and they should include explicit indications of authorship and sponsorship. A systematic review of 29 randomised controlled trials of patient decision aids found that they substantially increased patients' knowledge of problems, options and outcomes, achieved a reduction in the number of patients who were uncertain about what to do, reduced decisional conflict and increased participation in decision-making without increasing anxiety.[44]

When efforts are made to provide patients with unbiased evidence-based information about treatment options and likely outcomes, they usually make rational choices which are often more conservative and risk-adverse than those of the doctors in charge of their care. For example, American patients given full information about the pros and cons of prostate specific antigen (PSA) screening for prostate cancer were less likely to undergo the test than those who were not fully informed.[47] Prostatectomy rates fell when patients had the opportunity to view an interactive video programme outlining the risks and benefits of this surgical procedure[48], and similar findings are now emerging from a British trial of an information package for women referred for hysterectomy.[25] It seems that patients are often more risk-averse than the clinicians they consult.

Decision aids are not a substitute for good face-to-face communication between doctors and patients, but they can be a useful adjunct to the consultation. They have the potential to contribute to patient empowerment without increasing the burden on health professionals. Despite these well-researched attributes, good quality decision aids are still very scarce. Most of those that exist have been developed by academics for use in research studies. Meanwhile, patients continue to report considerable problems in getting hold of good quality information.

Dilemmas and tensions

The process of shared decision-making is complex. It has been suggested that a cooperative approach to choosing a treatment involves at least eight distinct skills or competences: [49]

1. Deciding how to involve the patient in the decision-making process.
2. Exploring their ideas about the problem.
3. Describing the treatment options.

4. Providing tailor-made information.
5. Checking that the patient understands the information and exploring their reactions.
6. Finding out the patient's preferred role in the decision-making process.
7. Making or deferring decisions.
8. Arranging follow-up.

The clinicians involved in drawing up this list felt it was feasible, though not necessarily easy, to go through each of these steps in a single consultation. However, successful resolution would depend on the willingness of both parties, doctor and patient, to engage in the process.

If both professionals and patients have access to the same information sources and both agree on the factors to be taken into account in deciding how to manage the problem, the quality and appropriateness of patient care could be considerably enhanced. If, on the other hand, they disagree on the approach or base their decisions on conflicting sources of information, the potential for conflict and mistrust will be increased. There are a variety of reasons why the relationship might become difficult:[50]

- The health care professional may feel threatened by a well informed or 'demanding' patient.
- Either or both parties may be misinformed because they are unable to discriminate between reliable and unreliable information or because they have misunderstood the information they have obtained.
- Patient and professional may make different interpretations of the same evidence.
- Either or both parties may be unwilling to share decision-making.
- Patients may be unsuccessful at communicating their preferences or professionals may not want to listen.
- Patients may be unwilling to accept external constraints imposed by the health system, e.g. time constraints, budgetary constraints, limitations on access, or on the availability of treatments.
- Either or both parties may be unwilling to accept responsibility for the cost consequences of their decisions and the potential knock-on effects on other patients.

Under English law patients have a legal right to refuse treatment, but they do not have a right to require a clinician to provide any treatment of their choice. Doctors cannot be forced to instigate treatment against their will, but unresolved disagreement could do serious damage to the therapeutic relationship and most clinicians will want to avoid it if at all possible. The clinician may therefore be tempted to concede to a patient's demands rather than risk a breakdown in the relationship. Alternatively the patient may give up the struggle to influence the treatment decision. Either way the outcome is likely to be unsatisfactory for at least one party if they continue to disagree and the therapeutic effect of the treatment may be diminished in the process.

It is tempting to think that this type of conflict might be resolved by resorting to the evidence. Evidence-based clinical guidelines, especially if they have the backing of nationally recognized organizations, could be helpful but they are not a panacea. Even the best scientific evidence gathered by the most rigorous methods has its limitations. It will often be insufficiently complete to provide guidance on what to do in every clinical situation and insufficiently reliable to eliminate the need for judgement. Expert opinion can vary when it comes to devising guidelines and the most careful consensus development procedures cannot rule out the possibility that different groups of experts will arrive at different conclusions after scrutinizing the same data. Patients may receive conflicting advice from different clinicians simply because clinicians' preferences vary. Many guidelines will be incomprehensible to patients because they were developed by, and for the use of, clinicians. Patients rarely have an input into guideline development and their perspectives may be completely absent from the evidence sources on which the guidelines are based.

Ethicists advise clinicians to challenge patients when the ethical principles of autonomy and justice collide, for example, if a patient wants a treatment that is not normally available and when providing it would result in depriving other patients of effective treatments.[51] In this situation it may be most appropriate to refuse to accede to the patient's choice. Individual autonomous choice cannot be the sole objective of a clinical encounter. We all exist in a social world and consideration has to be given to the effects of our actions and choices on others. However, as Ashcroft and colleagues have argued:

"Any ethical, and indeed any effective, approach to health care practice must be capable of recognizing the moral status of the choices of individual patients. Indeed this recognition must be central to such practice."[51]

If clinicians are to follow this advice they will need support and training on how to cope with conflict when it arises. They will also need more time. With average consultation times in UK general practice running at only eight minutes[52] and outpatient consultations being even shorter[53], it is hard to see how shared decision-making can be accommodated without a fundamental change in the organization of care. The informed patients of the future will almost certainly require more consultation time, not less, if their expectations are to be met.

Organisational support and training

Mere provision of good quality information and decision aids are necessary but not sufficient to engage patients in a more active role. For example, a set of ten leaflets designed to promote informed choice in pregnancy and childbirth was given to pregnant women in a randomised controlled trial in 13 maternity units in Wales.[54] Before the intervention about half of the women in both the intervention and the control units reported exercising informed choice in their maternity care. After the intervention this proportion increased slightly in both groups but there was no significant difference between the groups in the amount of change reported. An associated qualitative study explored the reasons for the lack of change.[55] Health professionals had been positive about the leaflets, but competing demands within the clinical environment had undermined their effective use. Time pressures meant there was limited opportunity for discussion of the options with patients and choice was often not available in practice. Fear of litigation tended to reinforce notions of "right" and "wrong" choices rather than informed choice. Hierarchical power structures meant that obstetricians tended to define the norms of clinical practice and hence which choices were possible. Pregnant women trusted the health professionals and rarely challenged the prevailing norms. Midwives failed to use the leaflets in an active way to initiate discussion with patients so their visibility as evidence based decision aids was greatly reduced. The authors concluded: "*the culture into which the leaflets were introduced supported existing normative patterns of care and this ensured informed compliance rather than informed choice.*"

Evidence that active use of decision aids can lead to a change in levels of involvement with consequences for treatment decisions comes from a three-arm trial of a decision aid for patients with menorrhagia.[25;56] The setting was six hospitals in south west England. An information package consisting of a booklet and an accompanying video were developed to help patients choose between surgical treatment (hysterectomy or endometrial ablation), drug therapy, a range of other possible interventions (e.g. dilation and curettage. removal of contraceptive coil, etc.) or no treatment. Just under 900 patients were randomised to receive the information package alone, the information package plus a structured interview with a nurse to help them think through their preferences, or standard care. Both interventions helped the women form treatment preferences and these tended to be more conservative than those of the group that did not receive the information package. Fewer women in both intervention groups wanted hysterectomy compared to the controls, but only those in the interview-plus-information-package group were significantly less likely to undergo hysterectomy. The nurse's role was important in helping women to get what they wanted. Those who had the information without the interview knew what they wanted, but they seemed less able to communicate their preference to the gynaecologist. An economic evaluation showed that the decision aid plus interview was a highly cost-effective intervention.

If health professionals find it difficult to support shared decision-making and informed choice, they will need training and support to implement a patient-centred approach.[57-60]. Training can make a significant difference. A recent systematic review found 17 trials of training interventions designed to promote patient-centred care in clinical consultations.[61] Outcomes measured included the quality of communication in the consultation, patient satisfaction, impact on health care behaviours such as compliance with medication and health-related behaviours (smoking, diet and exercise), health status and well-being. The review found fairly strong evidence that interventions to promote patient-centred care can lead to significant improvements in consultation processes and patient satisfaction. The impact on health status has not yet been demonstrated conclusively, but there are grounds for optimism because patients who are more actively engaged are more likely to follow treatment recommendations.

When patients are given the opportunity to make informed choices, they usually welcome it. Unreasonable or irrational demands are not as common as many clinicians fear. Patients often prefer more conservative and cheaper treatments than their doctors are inclined to recommend. Shared decision-making could be one of the best ways to ensure more appropriate use of health care resources, yet professional training programmes have been slow to incorporate it or to inculcate the necessary skills. Investment in decision aids has been confined to a few relatively small-scale initiatives. What is needed is a commitment to develop and disseminate good quality information and decision aids, coupled with staff training and organisational support. The effort and resources required are relatively modest, but the rewards for patients, clinicians and the health system as a whole could be considerable.

REFERENCES

[1] Tuckett D, Boulton M, Olson C, Williams A. Meetings between experts. London: Tavistock, 1985.

[2] Laine C,.Davidoff C. Patient centred medicine: a professional evolution. _Journal of the American Medical Association_ 1996;**275**:152–6.

[3] Coulter A,.Cleary PD. Patients' experiences with hospital care in five countries. _Health Affairs_ 2001;**20**:244–52.

[4] Grol R, Wensing M, Mainz J, Jung HP, Ferreira P, Hearnshaw H _et al._ Patients in Europe evaluate general practice care: an international comparison. _British Journal of General Practice_ 2000;**50**:882–7.

[5] Blanchard CG, Labrecque MS, Ruckdeschel JC, Blanchard EB. Information and decision-making preferences of hospitalized adult cancer patients. _Social Science and Medicine_ 1988;**27**:1139–45.

[6] Sutherland HJ, Llewellyn-Thomas HA, Lockwood GA, Tritchler DL, Till JE. Cancer patients: their desire for information and participation in treatment decisions. _Journal of the Royal Society of Medicine_ 1989;**82**:260–3.

[7] Savage R,.Armstrong D. Effect of a general practitioner's consulting style on patients' satisfaction. _British Medical Journal_ 1990;**301**:968–70.

[8] Coulter A. Quality of hospital care: measuring patients' experiences. _Proceedings of the Royal College of Physicians of Edinburgh_ 2001;**31**:34–6.

[9] Cassileth BR, Zupkis RV, Sutton-Smith K, March V. Information and participation preferences among cancer patients. _Annals of Internal Medicine_ 1980;**92**:832–6.

[10] Kennelly C,.Bowling A. Suffering in deference: a focus group study of older cardiac patients' preferences for treatment and perceptions of risk. _Quality in Health Care_ 2001;**10**(**Suppl. 1**): i23–i28.

[11] Krupat E, Rosenkranzz S L, Yeager C M, Barnard K, Putnam S M, and Inui, T. S. The practice orientations of physicians and patients: the effect of doctor-patient congruence on satisfaction. _Patient Education and Counseling_ 39, **49–59**. 2000.

[48] Wagner EH, Barrett P, Barry MJ, Barlow W, Fowler FJ. The effect of a shared decision making program on rates of surgery for benign prostatic hyperplasia: pilot results. *Medical Care* 1995;**33**:765–70.

[49] Elwyn G, Edwards A, Kinnersley P, Grol R. Shared decision making and the concept of equipoise: the competences of involving patients in healthcare choices. *British Journal of General Practice* 2000;**50**:892–9.

[50] Coulter A. The future. In Edwards A, Elwyn G, eds. *Evidence-based patient choice: inevitable or impossible?*, pp 308–21. Oxford: Oxford University Press, 2001.

[51] Ashcroft R, Hope T, Parker M. Ethical issues and evidence-based patient choice. In Edwards A, Elwyn G, eds. *Evidence-based patient choice: inevitable or impossible?*, pp 53–65. Oxford: Oxford University Press, 2001.

[52] Howie JGR, Heaney DJ, Maxwell M, Walker JJ, Freeman GK, Rai H. Quality at general practice consultations: cross sectional survey. *British Medical Journal* 1999;**319**:738–43.

[53] Waghorn A, McKee M. Surgical outpatient clinics: are we allowing enough time? *International Journal for Quality in Health Care* 1999;**11**:215–9.

[54] O'Cathain A, Walters SJ, Nicholl JP, Thomas KJ, Kirkham M. Use of evidence based leaflets to promote informed choice in maternity care: randomised controlled trial in everyday practice. *British Medical Journal* 2002;**324**:643–6.

[55] Stapleton H, Kirkham M, Thomas G. Qualitative study of evidence based leaflets in maternity care. *British Medical Journal* 2002;**324**:639–43.

[56] Kennedy ADM, Sculpher MJ, Coulter A, Dwyer N, Rees M, Abrams KR *et al.* Incorporating patients' preferences into clinical decision-making: a randomised controlled trial of decision aids in menorrhagia. *submitted* 2002.

[57] Elwyn G, Gwyn R, Edwards A, Grol R. Is 'shared decision-making' feasible in consultations for upper respiratory tract infections? Assessing the influence of antibiotic expectations using discourse analysis. *Health Expectations* 1999;**2**:105–17.

[58] Elwyn G, Edwards A, Gwyn R, Grol R. Towards a feasible model for shared decision making: focus group study with general practice registrars. *British Medical Journal* 1999;**319**:753–6.

[59] Stevenson FA, Barry CA, Britten N, Barber N, Bradley C. Doctor-patient communication about drugs: the evidence for shared decision making. *Social Science and Medicine* 2000;**50**:829–40.

[60] Towle A, Godolphin W. Framework for teaching and learning informed shared decision making. *British Medical Journal* 1999;**319**:766–9.

[61] Lewin SA, Skea ZC, Entwistle V, Zwarenstein M, Dick J. Interventions for providers to promote a patient centred approach in clinical consultations (Cochrane Review). Oxford: Update Software, 2002.

4. Managing care and ensuring safety: patient as care manager

"When doctors and patients consult with optimal efficiency, they become co-producers. In essence, consultations are not units of consumption, but units of production. Something has been created at the end of consultations, which was not present at their beginning: more and better understanding of patients' problems, of possible solutions, and of the personal circumstances in which these must be applied." [1]

Tudor Hart, J. Expectations of health care: promoted, managed or shared?
Health Expectations 1998

Enhancing self-efficacy

Most of us cope with minor illnesses without recourse to professional help. We go to the chemist or take ourselves off to bed when we have coughs, colds, flu, headaches, stomach pain or other minor problems which make us feel miserable but which we know are not dangerous and are probably self-limiting. If we do feel the need for advice, the doctor is not necessarily the first person we turn to. It is often forgotten that most healthcare is self-care. In looking after themselves and their family members lay people provide a far greater quantity of healthcare than do health professionals. Hannay used the metaphor of an iceberg to illustrate the point that health professionals, even those working in 'first contact' care such as general practice, see only a small fraction of the afflictions that could potentially trigger a consultation. [2] Some estimates have suggested that a majority of medical care (perhaps 85%) is self-care. [3]

There is a wealth of lay knowledge about illness and how to treat it and many people prefer to consult their family or friends before going to see a health professional. [4] Nevertheless, GPs often feel besieged by patients who don't really need their help. They report that a relatively high proportion of their daily consultations are for conditions that people could treat themselves. [5] There is a vicious cycle at work here. Struggling to cope with the large numbers of patients who queue in their surgeries every day, few GPs have the time, or perhaps the

52The Autonomous Patient

inclination, to help their patients to help themselves. Instead, by providing tests and prescriptions for minor everyday illnesses they reinforce the notion that doctor input is necessary, and in the process undermine patients confidence to cope with these problems themselves.

A variety of factors influence the decision to seek medical care, including ability to assess the problem and its severity, perceptions about the effectiveness of medical treatment, perceptions of one's own state of health, and feelings of confidence or self-efficacy. These perceptions are influenced by age, gender, educational level, cultural norms, social networks, co-morbidity and the attitudes of health care professionals. If health professionals act in a way which undermines people's coping skills, they can expect to see patients calling on their services with increasing frequency. On the other hand, if they could help their patients to help themselves they might be rewarded by fewer unnecessary consultations.

There is now a large body of evidence showing that educational interventions which enhance people's sense of self-efficacy can reduce the demand for medical intervention, leading to cost savings.[6,7] Studies have looked at the effects of training patients in specific behaviours and skills to manage their health problems. Conditions studied include arthritis, chronic pain, post-traumatic headache, myocardial infarction, seasickness, Parkinson's disease and hypertension. Beneficial effects have been demonstrated on various health outcomes, including blood pressure, reduced levels of depression, reduced pain, weight loss, and so on. A number of studies have found that these interventions can lead to reductions in the use of health services.

Recently policy makers concerned to secure best value for the resources expended on health care have taken a number of initiatives to capitalise on this knowledge. These have aimed to educate patients about when to seek professional help and when it is not necessary. The Doctor-Patient Partnership was set up with this aim and it was a main impetus behind the establishment of the government-funded telephone helpline, NHS Direct.[8,9] In its evaluation of NHS Direct, the National Audit Office concluded that the introduction of the telephone helpline has begun to reduce demands on out-of-hours services, albeit not dramatically, but this trend could increase as people get used to using the service.[10]

Evidence from elsewhere confirms that well-organised educational programmes can have an effect on health service utilisation. For example, a programme which distributed educational self-care manuals and a monthly newsletter to people living in Rhode Island, USA, resulted in statistically significant decreases of around 17% in ambulatory visit rates. Similar initiatives have been introduced in Idaho and in Oregon, with similar reported effects.[11;12] An American group, the Centre for Information Therapy, has been established to promote the idea that information can have a therapeutic role in helping patients to manage their symptoms or health problems. They are encouraging clinicians to offer an 'information therapy' prescription to the patient or carer at every clinic visit, for every medical test or surgical procedure, for every hospitalisation and for continuing care.[13]

Educational initiatives such as these are a good idea, but unless they are accompanied by a change in the way health professionals respond to patients they are unlikely to have a sustained impact. It is understandable that doctors are reluctant to challenge their patients about wasting their time, but failure to suggest self-help alternatives to medical treatment only perpetuates the problem. Reaching for the prescription pad because this appears to be what the patient wants rather than because a prescription is necessary only stores up problems for the future.[14] Unfortunately this is often the easiest and quickest way to end a consultation, but the net effect is to increase the total workload, thus compounding the problem.

Effective communication about medicines
Effective doctor-patient communication is critical to the delivery of appropriate health care. If patients beliefs and fears are not fully addressed in clinical consultations, there is a strong likelihood that problems will be missed and treatment may be ineffective. If the doctor does not understand the patient's attitude to taking medicines or does not adequately communicate the reasons for prescribing a particular drug, the patient may fail to take the prescription as recommended, reducing its efficacy. Patients want the doctor to listen to their concerns but failure to address the patient's agenda is a common occurrence.[15]

Most patients prefer to consult a sympathetic doctor interested in their worries and expectations, who discusses and agrees the problem and treatment.[16] This type of consulting style is more likely to foster the type of full information exchange necessary to reach an accurate diagnosis, but it will require longer consultations than is currently the norm.[17] Accurate diagnosis depends on taking a full history from the patient together with careful assessment of clinical signs and symptoms. If the patient's role is diminished, the likelihood of error is increased. Failure to institute appropriate management following receipt of test results could also be reduced if patients were encouraged to ask for explanations of these, but lack of clear explanations is a common complaint.[18]

The quality of clinical communication can have an effect on outcome.[19-21] Patients who are well informed about prognosis and treatment options, including benefits, harms and side-effects, are more likely to adhere to treatments, leading to better health outcomes.[22] They are also less likely to accept ineffective or risky procedures.[23-25] [24;25] Educational interventions to improve communication by increasing patients' participation in consultations have been shown to lead to improvements in functional status and physiological measures such as blood pressure and blood sugar control.[26]

Misunderstandings between patients and doctors about prescribing decisions are quite common.[27] The doctor may be unaware of relevant facts about the patient's medical history, for example, experience of side-effects or use of over-the-counter medicines; the patient may be unaware of the purpose of the prescription or the correct dose or the likelihood of side-effects; or the doctor may prescribe an unnecessary treatment which he thinks the patient wants, purely to preserve their relationship.

A detailed observational study of 62 general practice consultations in England found many failures in communication about prescribed medicines.[28] GPs frequently failed to give the patients the name of a newly prescribed medicine or details of the correct dosage, and they often omitted any mention of possible side-effects. They made assumptions about patients' preferences without checking these out, and patients were reluctant to tell the GP if they didn't want a prescription. GPs cited lack of time and other organisational pressures as barriers to sharing decisions, but they also expressed the belief that their patients lacked the will or ability to participate in treatment decision making.

This belief that patients cannot or do not want to be involved seriously impedes plans to promote more effective use of medicines based on the notion of *concordance.* Concordance is the model advocated by a working party established by the Royal Pharmaceutical Society of Great Britain.[29] They reviewed the literature on compliance and concluded that almost half of all patients who suffer from chronic diseases do not take their medication as recommended, resulting in huge personal and financial cost in avoidable continuing illness and premature death, as well as increased health expenditure. For example, a study of patients prescribed medication for high blood pressure found that about half dropped out of treatment altogether and about a third of those who continued to take the medication failed to take it in sufficient quantities to achieve a beneficial effect.[30]

While there may sometimes be practical or physiological reasons for not taking medicines in fully therapeutic doses, the working party concluded that the most salient and prevalent cause is the beliefs that people hold about their medication and about medicines in general. They argued that approaches adopted hitherto to improve rates of compliance by trying to persuade patients to 'follow doctor's orders' had fallen wide of the mark. Instead a different model of the relationship between patient and prescriber was required based on negotiation between equals in order to develop a therapeutic alliance. Concordance was defined as follows:

> "The clinical encounter is concerned with two sets of contrasted but equally cogent health beliefs – that of the patient and that of the doctor. The task of the patient is to convey her or his health beliefs to the doctor; and of the doctor to enable this to happen. The task of the doctor or other prescriber is to convey his or her (professionally informed) health beliefs to the patient; and of the patient, to entertain these. The intention is to assist the patient to make as informed a choice as possible about the diagnosis and treatment, about benefit and risk and to take full part in a therapeutic alliance. Although reciprocal, this is an alliance in which the most important determinants are agreed to be those that are made by the patient."[29]

This view of the problem has considerable support in the research literature.[31] Reasons for non-compliance can appear entirely rational when looked at from the patient's perspective. Patients often weigh up the pros and cons of taking the drugs, either consciously or unconsciously. Fear of side-effects is a significant factor, as is the time, effort and organisational skills involved, feelings of stigma related to being dependent on medicines, and so on. Failure to provide accurate comprehensible information to help patients quantify the risks and benefits of not taking medicines is an important cause of non-compliance. Patients who are given full information about the purpose of medicines and their likely effects, including side-effects, are more likely to take them as recommended, leading to better health outcomes.[32]

Achieving change will be no easy task though. A systematic review of 17 randomised controlled trials found that interventions involving various combinations of more convenient care, information, counselling, reminders, self-monitoring, reinforcement, family therapy and other forms of help could have a beneficial effect on compliance with prescribed medication.[33] But the authors of this review expressed surprise that a problem which is so important and which has major health and economic consequences has generated so few rigorous studies. It is equally surprising that so little attention has been given to implementing the lessons from the research that has been done. The barriers appear to be cultural rather than practical or financial.

Self-management of chronic disease
People with long-term health problems often become quite expert in managing their treatment and care and management of chronic diseases usually depends on patients playing an active role. For example, people with diabetes have to monitor their blood sugar levels and give themselves regular injections, people with asthma must become knowledgeable about inhalers and use them appropriately, and people on long-term medication must take their pills at regular intervals. We wouldn't expect health professionals to take on these responsibilities without education and training, but patients are usually expected to do it without such support. A survey carried out for the Audit Commission found that a significant proportion of people with diabetes did not understand about key elements of diabetes care.[34] When asked if their HbA1c had been measured in the past year, 40% of a national sample of 1,400 people with diabetes said they didn't know. Older people, those with type 2 diabetes, and ethnic minority respondents had particularly low levels of knowledge of how to care for themselves.

There is now a substantial body of evidence that shows that enhancing patients' role in self-management of chronic diseases and reducing dependence on health professionals can produce very beneficial results. Given appropriate training and clinical support when necessary, patients with long-term conditions can look after themselves most effectively and their quality of life can be much improved.

An example comes from some interesting work with arthritis patients carried out under the auspices of Arthritis Care. In the *Challenging Arthritis* programme patients are invited to attend training courses during which they learn the techniques of self-care, including use of medication, pain control methods, how to handle emotional, social and work problems, and how to monitor changes in symptoms and disease progression and take appropriate action. Reports from more than 70 studies of arthritis patient education suggest it can be effective in changing knowledge, health-related behaviour, psychosocial status and health status.[35]

A distinctive aspect of the arthritis self-management courses is that they are run by fellow sufferers. These volunteers are encouraged to act as facilitators rather than tutors. Using teaching methods based on Bandura's self-efficacy theory[36], participants learn strategies to enhance self-efficacy such as weekly action planning and feedback, how to reinterpret the causes of symptoms, different management techniques, group problem-solving, setting personal goals and monitoring progress. Rigorous evaluation of these training programmes in the US has shown that they succeeded in greatly increasing patients' knowledge, but more importantly patients reported improvements in symptom severity including levels of distress, fatigue, disability and ability to participate in everyday activities and they were less likely to be admitted to hospital.[37]

Similar educational programmes have been established for patients with a range of chronic diseases, including diabetes, chronic lung disease, heart disease, stroke, depression, chronic pain, insomnia, sickle cell disease and multiple sclerosis. A number of these programmes have been independently evaluated, with largely positive results. For example, studies have documented benefits for children and adults with asthma.[38;39] A systematic review of 22 randomised controlled trials of asthma self-management programmes found that they led to reduced hospitalisation rates, fewer emergency room visits, fewer unscheduled visits to the doctor, fewer days off work or school and fewer disturbed nights due to inability to sleep.[40] There is striking evidence that self-management programmes can be remarkably cost-effective. One self-management programme claimed savings of $11 in normal care for every $1 spent on the programme.[41]

This evidence of cost-effectiveness has attracted the attention of the Department of Health in England which has recently launched *The Expert Patient* initiative.[42] This initiative aims to promote the idea that patient expertise should be a central component in the management of chronic conditions. Patients organisations are being encouraged to develop patient-led self-management courses. The success of the programme must be judged against its impact on the lives of people with chronic diseases, including those who have difficulty in gaining access to services, for example people living in rural areas, people whose ethnicity, culture or language present barriers, and those with low education or literacy levels. The government is hoping that these attempts to promote self-care will result in considerable savings. A recent report for the Treasury cited estimates that for every £100 spent on encouraging self-care, around £150 worth of benefits could be delivered in return.[43] The new enthusiasm for self-care risks disappointment and disillusion if it is assumed that it will automatically lead to a dramatic reduction in demand for health services.[44] This certainly won't happen unless there is also a significant change in the way patients and professionals interact with each other.

Patient-held records
For years medical records have been seen as the property of the clinician, rather than the patient. Few patients have seen their notes and most are unaware of their right to do so. In both primary and secondary care, the notes are kept out of patients' reach wherever possible, and the way in which they are designed and used has reinforced the notion that they are for health professionals only. Referral letters and test results are often given to patients in sealed envelopes with no expectation that they will read or understand them. Curious patients are sometimes actively discouraged or reprimanded if they try to learn more about what has been recorded on their notes.

There are some exceptions to this general rule, however. Child health records are given to parents as a matter of course nowadays and patient-held records are relatively common in ante-natal care. A number of studies have examined the effects of giving patients access to their records.[45-48] In general these have found that patients are enthusiastic about holding their own notes. Holding the records and reading them can increase patients' knowledge of their health state and their sense of shared responsibility for their own health care. On the other hand, health professionals' attitudes to patient-held records are often ambivalent: while welcoming the idea in theory, the practical obstacles are often deemed insurmountable.[49]

The difficulties might seem even more problematic in the case of computer-based records. Yet experiments in giving patients access to computerised records have produced very positive results.[50;51] One British general practice discovered errors in more than 30% of medical records when patients were encouraged to review their notes.[51]

If patients were encouraged to review their notes and provided with clear explanations of the meaning of the clinical terms used, it could be very empowering. If this was to become common practice it could have a beneficial effect on the clarity of communications between staff as well. Knowing that records will be read by patients might affect what health professionals choose to record, but if it improves the clarity of note writing it could enhance communications between multi-disciplinary teams. Above all it has the potential to change the dynamics of the relationship between patients and health professionals in fairly fundamental ways.

Patient safety

Patients are usually thought of in a passive way as the victims of errors and safety failures, but there is considerable scope for them to play an active part in ensuring their care is effective and appropriate, in preventing mistakes and assuring their own safety. The patient is, or should be, involved in helping to reach an accurate diagnosis; choosing an appropriate treatment or management strategy; choosing a suitably experienced and safe provider; ensuring that treatment is appropriately administered, monitored and adhered to; and identifying side-effects or adverse events quickly and taking appropriate action.

Diagnostic accuracy depends on good communication. Failure to listen to what the patient is saying about his/her symptoms, or dismissing their concerns too hastily, can lead to misdiagnosis. With GP consultations lasting only eight minutes or so, it is often difficult for the patient to get across all the information they feel is important. The national survey of general practice patients carried out in 1998 revealed that patients didn't always feel listened to by their GPs. Only 60% of those surveyed reported that their GP always listened to them and only 51% felt their GP always took their opinions seriously.[52] Patients' sense of 'enablement' seems to be enhanced by longer GP consultations and better continuity of care.[53] Safety is more likely to be compromised if consultations are rushed.

Patients who know what to expect in relation to quality standards can check on appropriate performance of clinical tasks. The Foundation for Accountability in the USA promotes consumer information about evidence-based care so that patients know what should happen during the course of an illness. For example, patients with diabetes are encouraged to check that they receive regular blood tests, regular retinal and foot examinations, and advice on how to quit smoking.[54] If patients had access to clinical guidelines (or patient versions of these), they could ensure that their care was compliant with recommended standards.

Prescribing errors are relatively common.[55] These include administration of drugs or dosages which are inappropriate for the patient because of contra-indications or unnoticed adverse reactions, failure to communicate essential information, and errors in transcribing medical records. Many of these errors could be avoided if communication with patients was improved and they were encouraged to speak up when they notice unexplained changes in their medication. Schemes which rely on doctors to report suspected adverse reactions to medicines suffer from widespread under-reporting.[56;57] These could be enhanced if patients were encouraged to report adverse events directly to a central scheme. Such a scheme has existed in Sweden for the past 25 years. Operated by KILEN, the Consumer Institute for Medicines and Health, the project provides reporting forms to patients who wish to report adverse reactions to medicines.[58] The submitted forms are entered onto a database which is analysed and reports submitted to relevant government agencies. In the US patients can report adverse reactions directly to the Food and Drug Administration if they wish. The UK Consumers Association is now calling for the establishment of a similar scheme in Britain.[59]

Patients undergoing surgical operations should be encouraged to report post-surgical complications promptly so that swift action can be taken if necessary. Unfortunately, lack of information about what to watch out for after discharge from hospital is a very common complaint. In a postal survey of patients discharged from hospital, 31% of respondents said they weren't given clear explanations of the results of their surgical procedures, 60% weren't given sufficient information about danger signals to watch out for at home after discharge from hospital, and 61% weren't told when they could resume their normal activities.[18] If greater attention was paid to providing this type of information, it could lead to a reduction in the rate of complications and readmissions.

Sensitive communication is also essential if mistakes or adverse events occur. Patients who are victims of medical errors often suffer considerable psychological trauma, both as a result of the original incident and through the way the incident is managed. If a medical injury occurs it is important to listen to the patient and/or their family, acknowledge the damage, give an honest and open explanation and an apology, ask about emotional trauma and anxieties about future treatment, and provide practical and financial help quickly.[60] Unfortunately this doesn't always happen. A survey of 227 litigants to examine their reasons for taking legal action against their health care providers found that the overwhelming majority were dissatisfied with the nature and clarity of the explanations they were given and the lack of sympathy displayed by staff after the incident.[61] In some cases litigation might have been avoided altogether if staff had dealt with patients more sensitively.

Responsible patients
At most stages of patient care there is potential for patients to contribute through provision of diagnostic information and by participation in treatment decisions, choice of provider, management and treatment of disease and monitoring adverse events. This requires that healthcare professionals encourage and support a more active stance from patients, but also that patients are prepared, where possible, to take more responsibility for their health and their care.

Honest information, clear, supportive communication and a participative approach should be the watchwords in promoting effective management and safe care. These principles apply at all levels of health policy, including the one-to-one encounter in the clinic, the publication of information about quality standards and outcomes among providers, the provision of government advice on public health risks, and the way in which the consequences of mistakes and adverse events are dealt with when they occur. Patients and citizens have a legitimate interest in, and responsibility for, their own safety. It is incumbent on providers and policy makers to take active steps to involve them in efforts to improve the quality and safety of medical care.

REFERENCES

[1] Tudor Hart J. Expectations of health care: promoted, managed or shared? *Health Expectations* 1998;**1**:1–2.

[2] Hannay DR. The symptom iceberg – a study of community health. London: Routledge and Kegan Paul, 1979.

[3] Vickery DM, Kalmer H, Lowry D, Constantine M, Wright E, Loren W. Effect of a self-care education program on medical visits. *Journal of the American Medical Association* 1983;**250**:2952–6.

[4] Popay J,.Williams G. Public health research and lay knowledge. *Social Science and Medicine* 1996;**42**:759–68.

[5] Dunnell K, Cartwright A. Medicine takers, prescribers and hoarders. London: 1972.

[6] Vickery DM,.Lynch WD. Demand management: enabling patients to use medical care appropriately. *Journal of Occupational and Environmental Medicine* 1995;**37**:551–7.

[7] Crow, R., Gage, H., Hampson, S., Hart, J., Kimber, A., and Thomas, H. The role of expectancies in the placebo effect and their use in the delivery of health care: a systematic review. 1999. Southampton, Health Technology Assessment, NHS R&D HTA Programme.

[8] Doctor Patient Partnership. www.doctorpatient.org . 2002.

[9] NHS Direct. www.nhsdirect.nhs.uk . 2002.

[10] Comptroller and Auditor General. NHS Direct in England. HC505. 25-1–2002. London, The Stationery Office.

[11] Kemper DW. Healthwise Handbook. Boise, Idaho: Healthwise Inc., 1997.

[12] Kieschnick T, Adler LJ, Jimison HB. Health informatics directory. Baltimore: Williams and Wilkins, 2002.

[13] Centre for Information Therapy. www.informationtherapy.org . 2002.

[14] Cockburn J,.Pit S. Prescribing behaviour in clinical practice: patients' expectations and doctors' perceptions of patients' expectations – a questionnaire study. *British Medical Journal* 1997;**315**:520–3.

[15] Barry CA, Bradley CP, Britten N, Stevenson FA, Barber N. Patients' unvoiced agendas in general practice consultations: qualitative study. *British Medical Journal* 2000;**320**:1246–50.

[16] Little P, Everitt H, Williamson I, Warner G, Moore M, Gould C *et al.* Observational study of effect of patient centredness and positive approach on outcomes of general practice consultations. *British Medical Journal* 2001;**323**:908–11.

[17] Campbell SM, Hann M, Hacker J, Burns C, Oliver D, Thapar A *et al.* Identifying predictors of high quality care in English general practice: observational study. *British Medical Journal* 2001;**323**:784–7.

[18] Coulter A. Quality of hospital care: measuring patients' experiences. *Proceedings of the Royal College of Physicians of Edinburgh* 2001;**31**:34–6.

[19] Stewart MA. Effective physician-patient communication and health outcomes: a review. *Canadian Medical Association Journal* 1995;**152**:1423–33.

[20] Di Blasi Z, Harkness E, Ernst E, Georgiou A, Kleijnen J. Influence of context effects on health outcomes: a systematic review. *Lancet* 2001;**357**:757–62.

[21] Simpson M, Buckman R, Stewart M, Maguire P, Lipkin M, Novack D *et al*. Doctor-patient communication: the Toronto consensus statement. *British Medical Journal* 1991;**303**:1385–7.

[22] Mullen PD. Compliance becomes concordance. *British Medical Journal* 1997;**314**:691.

[23] Flood AB, Wennberg JE, Nease RF, Fowler FJ, Ding J, Hynes LM. The importance of patient preference in the decision to screen for prostate cancer. *Journal of General Internal Medicine* 1996;**11**:342–9.

[24] Wagner EH, Barrett P, Barry MJ, Barlow W, Fowler FJ. The effect of a shared decision making program on rates of surgery for benign prostatic hyperplasia: pilot results. *Medical Care* 1995;**33**:765–70.

[25] Wolf AMD, Nasser JF, Wolf AM, Schorling JB. The impact of informed consent on patient interest in prostate-specific antigen screening. *Archives of Internal Medicine* 1996;**156**:1333 6.

[26] Kaplan SH, Greenfield S, Ware JE. Assessing the effects of physician-patient interactions on the outcomes of chronic disease. *Medical Care* 1989;**27**:S110–S127.

[27] Britten N, Stevenson FA, Barry CA, Barber N, Bradley CP. Misunderstandings in prescribing decisions in general practice: qualitative study. *British Medical Journal* 2000;**320**:484–8.

[28] Stevenson FA, Barry CA, Britten N, Barber N, Bradley C. Doctor-patient communication about drugs: the evidence for shared decision making. *Social Science and Medicine* 2000;**50**:829–40.

[29] Marinker, M and *et al*. From compliance to concordance: achieving shared goals in medicine taking. 1997. London, Royal Pharmaceutical Society of Great Britain.

[30] Dunbar-Jacob J, Dwyer K, Dunning EJ. Compliance with anti-hypertensive regimen: a review of the research in the 1980s. *Annals of Behavioural Medicine* 1991;**13**:31–9.

[31] Donovan JL,.Blake DR. Patient non-compliance: deviance or reasoned decision-making? *Social Science and Medicine* 1992;**34**:507–13.

[32] Lowe CJ, Raynor DK, Courtney EA, Purvis J, Teale C. Effects of self medication programme on knowledge of drugs and compliance with treatment in elderly patients. *British Medical Journal* 1995;**310**:1229–31.

[33] Haynes, R. B., Montague, P., Oliver, T., McKibbon, K. A., Brouwers, M. C., and Kanani, R. Interventions for helping patients to follow prescriptions for medications (Cochrane Review). Cochrane Library (4). 2000. Oxford: Update Software.

[34] Raleigh VS,.Clifford GM. Knowledge, perceptions and care of people with diabetes in England and Wales. Journal of Diabetes Nursing 2002;**6(3)**:72–8.

[35] Lorig K, Konkol L, Gonzalez V. Arthritis patient education: a review of the literature. *Patient Education and Counseling* 1987;**10**:208–52.

[36] Bandura A. Self-efficacy: toward a unifying theory of behavioral change. *Psychological Review* 1977;**84**:191.

[37] Lorig, K. R, Sobel, D. S, Stewart, A. L., Brown, B. W., Bandura, A., Ritter, P, Gonzalex, V. M., Laurent, D. D., and Holman, H. R. Evidence suggesting that a chronic disease self-management program can improve health status while reducing hospitalization. *Medical Care* 37, **5–14**. 1999.

[38] Gebert N, Hummelink R, Konning J, Staab D, Schmidt S, Szczepanski R *et al*. Efficacy of a self-management program for childhood asthma - a prospective controlled study. *Patient Education and Counseling* 1998;**35**:213-20.

[39] Lahdensuo A, Haahtela T, Herrala J, Kava T, Kiviranta K, Kuusisto P *et al*. Randomised comparison of guided self management and traditional treatment of asthma over one year. *British Medical Journal* 1996;**312**:748-52.

[40] Gibson, P. G., Coughlan, J., Wilson, A. J., Abramson, M., Bauman, A., Hensley, M. J., and Walters, E. H. Self-management education and regular practitioner review for adults with asthma (Cochrane Review). The Cochrane Library (Issue 4). 2000. Update Software.

[41] Lahdensuo A. Guided self management of asthma – how to do it. *British Medical Journal* 1999;**319**:759–60.

[42] Department of Health. The Expert Patient: a new approach to chronic disease management for the 21st century. 2001. London, Department of Health.

[43] Wanless, D. Securing our future health: taking a long-term view (final report). 2002. London, HM Treasury.

[44] Rogers A, Hassell K, Nicolaas G. Demanding patients? Analysing the use of primary care. Buckingham: Open University Press, 1999.

[45] Elbourne D, Richardson M, Chalmers I, *et al*. The Newbury Maternity Care Study: a randomised controlled trial to evaluate a policy of women holding their own obstetric records. *British Journal of Obstetrics and Gynaecology* 1987;**94**:612–9.

[46] Lovell A, Zander LJ, James CE, *et al*. The St. Thomas's maternity case notes study: a randomised controlled trial to assess the effects of giving expectant mothers their own maternity case notes. *Paediatric Perinatal Epidemiology* 1987;**1**:57–66.

[47] Essex B, Doig R, Renshaw J. Pilot study of records of shared care for people with mental illnesses. *British Medical Journal* 1990;**300**:1442–6.

[48] Drury M, Yudkin P, Harcourt J, Fitzpatrick R, Jones L, Alcock C *et al*. Patients with cancer holding their own records: a randomised controlled trial. *British Journal of General Practice* 2000;**50**:105–10.

[49] Ayana M, Pound P, Ebrahim S. The views of therapists on the use of a patient-held record in the care of stroke patients. *Clinical rehabilitation* 1998;**12**:328–37.

[50] Jones R, Pearson J, McGregor S, Cawsey AJ, Barrett A, Craig N *et al*. Randomised trial of personalised computer based information for cancer patients. *British Medical Journal* 1999;**319**:1241–7.

[51] Pyper, C., Amery, J., Watson, M., Thomas, B., and Crook, C. ERDIP online patient access project. 2001. Oxford, Bury Knowle Health Centre.

[52] Department of Health. National survey of NHS patients: general practice 1998. Airey, C. and Erens, B. 2002. London, Department of Health.

[53] Howie JGR, Heaney DJ, Maxwell M, Walker JJ, Freeman GK, Rai H. Quality at general practice consultations: cross sectional survey. *British Medical Journal* 1999;**319**:738–43.

[54] Foundation for Accountability. www.facct.org . 2002.

[55] Dean B, Barber N, Schachter M. What is a prescribing error? *Quality in Health Care* 2000;**9**:232–7.

[56] Moride Y, Haramburu F, Requejo AA, *et al*. Under-reporting of adverse drug reactions in general practice. *British Journal of Clinical Pharmacology* 1997;**43**:177–81.

[57] Smith CC, Bennett PM, Pearce HM, et al. Adverse drug reactions in a hospital medical unit meriting notification to the Committee on Safety of Medicines. *British Journal of Clinical Pharmacology* 2002;**42**:423–9.

[58] KILEN. www.kilen.org . 2002.

[59] Anon. Drug side effects. Health Which (April). 2001.

[60] Vincent C,.Coulter A. Patient safety: what about the patient? *Quality and Safety in Health Care* 2002;**11**:76–80.

[61] Vincent C, Young M, Phillips A. Why do people sue doctors? A study of patients and relatives taking legal action. *Lancet* 1994;**343**:1609–13.

5. Assessing and improving health care delivery: patient as evaluator

"These days virtually every health organization is knee-deep in 'redesign'. Few, however, invite patients to join in such efforts..... Efforts to improve care might take strikingly different shape if patients worked as full partners with health professionals to design and implement change."[1]

Delbanco, T. et al. Healthcare in a land called PeoplePower: nothing about me without me. Health Expectations 2001

Feedback from patients

There are many views and perspectives on what constitutes high quality health care.[2] Quality from the *professional* perspective includes adherence to professional standards, ensuring technical competencies, achieving desired outcomes and striving to expand medical knowledge. Quality from a *management* perspective incorporates factors such as appropriate use of resources, ensuring high quality care, identifying and managing risks, and facilitating service developments. Quality from a *patient* perspective typically includes access, responsiveness, good communication, clear information provision, appropriate treatment, relief of symptoms and improvement in health status. Ensuring that treatment is appropriate and clinically effective requires attention to patients' subjective experiences as well as to the technical aspects of care.

Research with hospital patients has shown how traumatic the experience of hospitalisation can be.[3] They describe a sense of powerlessness, a loss of dignity and a feeling of vulnerability. Having to wait a long time before being allocated a bed can be upsetting and humiliating. It can also be distressing to be moved from ward to ward. Most patients make very positive comments about the clinical staff who care for them, but they complain of being asked the same questions over and over again, especially during ward rounds which can be an intimidating experience. They often find it difficult to get clear answers to their questions, and sometimes receive contradictory information from different members of staff.

Pain control is not always handled well and test results are not always reported back to patients, particularly negative results, resulting in needless anxiety. Patients are often not told the name of the person who is in charge of their care and discharge arrangements are sometimes poorly coordinated, leaving patients feeling disempowered just at the time when they need to feel confident to take charge of their own care at home.

General practice care is usually much less traumatic than hospital and patients' evaluations tend to be more positive, but studies of their experiences reveal plenty of scope for improvement, for example in access arrangements, communication skills, information exchange and education for patients.[4] Health care staff are often unaware of patients' concerns. When you have spent much of your working life in a hospital or other health care facility it can be hard to imagine what it feels like to be a patient there, unfamiliar with the routines, unsure what is likely to happen to you and anxious because you are ill. Systematic feedback in the form of regular patient surveys can help staff to see things through the eyes of the patient enabling them to centre quality improvement efforts on their needs and wishes. Patients are in a good position to evaluate the quality of their care and it is increasingly being recognised that patient feedback ought to be a central part of any quality improvement programme. Feedback can help refocus the attention of clinicians and managers on the patient's experience and can galvanise them into action to improve quality standards.

Patient satisfaction

The main way in which patients' views on health care performance have traditionally been sought is through the measurement of patient satisfaction. Satisfaction is not usually recorded routinely in health care so specially designed surveys have to be organised to seek the views of representative samples of patients or members of the public. There are at least five levels of aggregation at which these views may be relevant: (1) satisfaction with the functioning of the health system as a whole; (2) satisfaction with care provided in specific organisations, for example hospitals or general practices; (3) satisfaction with care provided by particular specialties or hospital departments; (4) satisfaction with the performance of individual clinicians, and (5) satisfaction with the outcomes of specific treatments.

Satisfaction is an ill-defined concept which has been measured in many different ways.[5-9] Generally recognised as multi-dimensional in nature, there is no consensus on which domains should be included or which are most important. Patient satisfaction is sometimes treated as an outcome measure, i.e. satisfaction with health status following treatment, and sometimes as a process measure, i.e. satisfaction with the way in which care was delivered. Satisfaction ratings reflect three variables: the personal preferences of the patient, the patient's expectations, and the realities of the care received. Public attitudes are influenced by many factors including the media, commercial pressures and by patients' interaction with health professionals. Expectations may also be influenced by cultural norms and by health status. Disentangling the effects of expectations, experience and satisfaction is a major problem when patients' views are used to measure performance. Studies have found systematic differences between the views of the public (healthy people/potential patients) and the views of current users of health services. Patients may be further differentiated in terms of disease severity, chronic versus acute, and so on. Expectations and concerns are likely to be affected by the patient's experience of health care and their knowledge of, or dependency on, health care providers.

Health care providers in Europe and the USA have been measuring patient satisfaction for many years, but often these surveys have been conceptually flawed and methodologically weak.[10] They have tended to focus on managers' or clinicians' agendas rather than on the topics which are most important to patients and they are frequently too 'broad brush' to produce actionable results. The complexities of modern health care and the diversity of patients' expectations and experiences cannot be reliably evaluated by asking global rating questions such as "How satisfied were you with your care in hospital X?" nor by focusing solely on food and amenities while ignoring patients' concerns about their illness and clinical care. Typically such surveys elicit overwhelmingly positive ratings which do not reflect reported experience. Patient surveys have often been used simply as marketing tools, with providers making claims on the basis of poorly designed and badly conducted surveys that "95% of our patients are satisfied".

Measuring patients' experience
More rigorous methods are required if quality improvement efforts are to become truly patient-centred. The critiques of patient satisfaction surveys have

led to a new emphasis on measuring patients' experience rather than satisfaction. Instead of asking patients to rate their care on a Likert scale (e.g. excellent, very good, good, fair, poor), a more valid approach is to ask patients to report in detail on their experiences by asking them specific questions about whether or not certain processes and events occurred during the course of a specific episode of care.[11] Building on extensive qualitative research to determine which aspects of care are important to patients, standardised instruments have been developed to measure the quality of care in relation to particular domains.[12]

The advantage of asking specific factual questions about detailed aspects of patients' experience is that answers to such questions are easier to interpret than the rating questions commonly included in patient satisfaction surveys. Knowing that, say, 15% of your patients rated their care as "fair" or "poor" doesn't give a manager or clinician much clue about what they need to do to improve the quality of care in their hospital. On the other hand, knowing more precise details of what went wrong, for example, the proportion of patients who felt they had to wait too long for the call button to be answered, and monitoring trends in these indicators over time, can be much more useful. Focusing on the details of patients' experience can help to pinpoint the problems much more precisely.

Instruments to measure patients' experience were developed by researchers at Harvard Medical School with funds from the Picker/Commonwealth Program for Patient-Centred Care, a programme established in 1987 under the auspices of the Commonwealth Fund of New York.[13] The aim was to explore patients' needs and concerns as patients themselves define them.[14] The Harvard team designed a patient feedback programme derived from qualitative research designed to find out what patients value about the experience of receiving health care and what they considered unacceptable.[11,15] They conducted focus groups with patients and their family members, reviewed the literature and consulted with health care professionals to determine key priorities.

This research programme resulted in the development of survey instruments designed to elicit reports from patients about concrete aspects of their experience. The first national survey using this tool involved telephone interviews with 6,000 recently hospitalised patients randomly selected from sixty-two hospitals in the USA, along with 2,000 of the friends or family members who served as their carers.[16;17] The Picker adult inpatient questionnaire has subsequently been used with many patients in the USA and elsewhere, including Australia, Canada and various European countries.[18-22]

Although these measures of patient-centred care are exclusively concerned with the process of care, there is evidence that patient-centredness measured in this way is associated with greater satisfaction and better health outcomes, including reductions in physical symptoms, complications and mortality rates. A study of 52 hospital units in south-eastern Michigan found that patients treated in hospital units that performed best on the Picker measures (i.e. had low problem scores) had significantly better outcomes (complications and unexpected deaths) than those that were less patient-centred. However, patient-centred care does not come cheap – costs were higher in the better performing units.[23] Another study obtained completed questionnaires from 762 patients treated for acute myocardial infarction (AMI) in 23 New Hampshire hospitals. After adjustment for post-discharge health status and other clinical factors, patients experiencing worse hospital care as measured by the Picker instrument had lower ratings of overall health and physical health and were more likely to have chest pain after AMI than other patients.[24]

Nowadays the survey is usually administered by mail rather than by telephone. This approach to measuring patients' experience has since been adopted for use in the Consumer Assessment of Health Plans (CAHPS) surveys in the USA, the WHO responsiveness surveys and the national NHS patient survey programme in England.[25-27] The Picker Institute, which was established by the team who developed this new approach to measuring patients' experience, has extensive experience of organising surveys of patients' experience of health care in different countries. Picker surveys have been used since 1987 in hospitals in the USA and since 1997 in Germany, Sweden, Switzerland and the UK. A recent study compared patients' experience in the five countries.[21] The results are shown in Table 5:1 which gives the proportion of patients reporting a problem in relation to each of the items in the questionnaire. These 'problem scores' are then grouped into dimensions of patient experience, and the table shows the mean 'dimension score' for each country.

TABLE 5:1

Picker surveys of hospital inpatients: problem scores (%) and dimension scores (%) for hospitals in five countries (age and sex adjusted rates)[62]

	Switzerland	Germany	Sweden	USA	UK
	7,163 patients in 9 hospitals	2,663 patients in 6 hospitals	3,274 patients in 9 hospitals	47,576 patients in 272 hospitals	2,249 patients in 6 hospitals
Information and education					
Insufficient inform-ation in A&E	28.3	32.4	25.8	39.7	52.3
Delay to go to ward not explained	7.6	7.4	9.6	9.9	5.7
Doctors answers to questions not clear	10.7	17.1	21.9	21.2	27.7
Nurses answers to questions not clear	10.6	12.9	15.7	28.9	23.6
Test results not clearly explained	26.2	32.1	44.0	26.2	34.0
Dimension score	**16.7**	**20.4**	**23.4**	**25.2**	**28.7**
Coordination of care					
Emergency care not well organized*	18.6	20.5	N/a	26.4	37.0
Admission process not well organized*	15.3	23.4	N/a	21.2	20.1
Long wait to go to ward	13.0	18.0	28.6	26.8	15.0
No doctor in overall charge of care	7.1	10.4	28.8	11.4	15.1
Staff gave conflict-ing information	13.6	14.6	19.1	18.0	22.9
Scheduled tests or procedures not done on time	10.7	16.7	16.7	26.3	21.4
Dimension score	**13.1**	**17.2**	**N/a**	**21.7**	**21.9**

* Questions not included in Swedish surveys

continued

	Switzerland	Germany	Sweden	USA	UK
	7,163 patients in 9 hospitals	2,663 patients in 6 hospitals	3,274 patients in 9 hospitals	47,576 patients in 272 hospitals	2,249 patients in 6 hospitals
Physical comfort					
Didn't get help to go to bathroom/toilet	5.5	4.4	5.0	20.3	15.0
Had to wait too long after pressing call button	0.6	0.6	0.4	4.1	0.9
Had to wait too long for pain medicine	0.8	14.8	2.1	3.9	4.5
Staff did not do enough to control pain	4.9	11.4	8.9	16.2	14.6
Given too little pain medicine	1.1	2.4	3.7	5.9	6.5
Dimension score	**2.6**	**6.7**	**4.0**	**10.1**	**8.3**
Emotional support					
Doctor didn't discuss anxieties or fears	17.3	23.4	36.2	23.7	34.1
Didn't always have confidence in doctors	10.4	19.1	19.7	15.8	18.7
Nurse didn't discuss anxieties or fears	18.5	25.8	31.0	32.4	32.3
Didn't always have confidence in nurses	10.2	13.2	13.9	28.6	19.8
Not easy to find someone to talk to about concerns	17.1	28.0	29.0	33.7	30.3
Dimension score	**14.7**	**21.9**	**26.0**	**26.8**	**27.1**

continued

	Switzerland	*Germany*	*Sweden*	*USA*	*UK*
	7,163 patients in 9 hospitals	2,663 patients in 6 hospitals	3,274 patients in 9 hospitals	47,576 patients in 272 hospitals	2,249 patients in 6 hospitals
Respect for patients' preferences					
Doctors some-times talked as if I wasn't there	11.3	10.0	13.0	12.5	29.4
Nurses some-times talked as if I wasn't there	7.0	3.2	5.8	12.8	14.6
Didn't have enough say about treatment	35.7	46.1	53.8	37.0	59.4
Not always treated with respect and dignity	8.4	12.3	12.3	17.4	19.5
Dimension score	**15.6**	**17.9**	**21.2**	**19.9**	**30.7**
Involvement of family and friends					
Family didn't get opportunity to talk to doctor	13.8	17.0	13.8	22.8	32.3
Family not given enough info about condition	3.9	5.2	7.5	9.3	11.6
Family not given info needed to help recovery	16.9	27.6	22.4	25.9	38.5
Dimension score	**11.5**	**16.6**	**14.6**	**19.3**	**27.5**

continued

	Switzerland	Germany	Sweden	USA	UK
	7,163 patients in 9 hospitals	2,663 patients in 6 hospitals	3,274 patients in 9 hospitals	47,576 patients in 272 hospitals	2,249 patients in 6 hospitals
Continuity and transition					
Purpose of medicines not fully explained	13.1	23.3	18.9	14.8	23.1
Not told about medication side effects	36.1	43.7	51.3	31.5	36.0
Not told about danger signals to watch for at home	33.5	43.9	47.7	32.3	60.3
Not told when to resume normal activities	37.3	51.5	43.0	35.2	60.9
Dimension score	**30.0**	**40.6**	**40.2**	**28.4**	**45.1**
Overall impression					
Courtesy of admissions staff not good	2.7	4.4	6.1	5.7	2.5
Courtesy of doctors not good	2.8	6.1	8.4	4.7	6.9
Availability of doctors not good	3.8	5.3	27.3	11.9	30.0
Courtesy of nurses not good	2.6	4.9	4.4	7.6	5.6
Availability of nurses not good	1.5	2.3	16.3	14.1	29.8
Doctor/nurse teamwork not good*	3.9	6.1	n/a	7.5	8.1

continued

	Switzerland	Germany	Sweden	USA	UK
	7,163 patients in 9 hospitals	2,663 patients in 6 hospitals	3,274 patients in 9 hospitals	47,576 patients in 272 hospitals	2,249 patients in 6 hospitals
Overall rating of care "fair" or "poor"	3.7	6.6	7.4	8.1	8.5
Would not recommend this hospital to friends/family	3.6	5.0	2.8	4.8	7.8

In many cases the level of reported problems was high. For example, inadequate post-discharge information was a significant problem in each of the countries. More than a third of surgical patients in all countries felt inadequately prepared for how they would feel after the operation. Patients were also concerned about organisational issues, such as coordination of their care and delays in accessing tests and treatment, but these topics received fewer complaints on the whole. The questions which asked patients to give ratings of their overall impressions tended to receive quite favourable responses illustrating the point made above that general rating questions tend to mask the problems.

In all countries the most commonly reported problems concerned communications about clinical issues:

- didn't have enough say about treatment;
- insufficient information in emergency room;
- tests results not clearly explained;
- not told about medication side-effects;
- not told accurately how could feel after surgery;
- not told about danger signals to watch for at home; and
- not told when to resume normal activities.

These results offer compelling evidence that, in general, patients have unacceptably high rates of problems with selected issues, such as emergency care, explanations of test results and treatment options, opportunity to discuss anxieties with doctors or nurses and to have a say in their treatment, and information about treatment outcomes and follow-up care (e.g. after surgery or discharge from hospital). In the face of the common perception that patients' concerns centre on waiting times and hospitals' 'hotel' facilities, it is important to note that these survey results indicate greatest concern about clinical issues.

The difficulties of interpreting international comparisons are well known.[28] When considering these data, it is important to be aware of demographic differences, translation problems, cultural and health system differences. Nevertheless, the differences between the countries are very suggestive. Swiss patients reported markedly fewer problems than those in the other countries, producing the lowest (best) dimension scores for all except the continuity and transition dimension in which the US had the lowest score. The UK sample produced the worst scores on every dimension except physical comfort. Health care is much better resourced in Switzerland than in the UK. Patients in the UK and Sweden were more likely to report problems due to staff shortages than those in the other countries, probably reflecting the differences in resource levels.

Patient satisfaction is determined by expectations. The Picker surveys of patients' experience aim to collect factual reports of processes and events and are, arguably, less subject to variations in expectations. Nevertheless, it is possible that patients' views of appropriate care could differ substantially among the countries studied. However, those involved in the development of these surveys have verified that the questions asked are salient and important in each of the countries studied. Furthermore, a recent study in the UK, Norway, Sweden, Denmark, the Netherlands, Germany, Portugal, and Israel found that although patients in different cultures and health care systems have different views on certain aspects of care, many expectations and values are very similar, particularly with respect to doctor-patient communication and accessibility of services.[29]

Using patient feedback for quality improvement

Patient feedback surveys such as these provide a snapshot of the quality of care through the patient's eyes which can be used as the first step in a change programme. The findings can be used to prioritise areas where improvement is needed. Comparison against national and international benchmarks can be helpful for persuading staff that better care is possible. Studying survey results over time within one hospital can be a useful way of monitoring the effectiveness of quality improvement initiatives. Further examination of the procedures and processes used in different hospitals could provide useful insights on how to improve certain aspects of care.

Until recently, attempts to understand the patient's perspective on care depended on the efforts of a few enthusiasts. In hospitals or other care facilities where there was strong leadership and committed staff, there have been good examples of improvements as a direct result of feeding back results from surveys documenting patients' experience. For example, the Beth Israel Hospital in Boston used regular patient surveys to identify the need to improve the quality of their discharge planning process, particularly in patient education.[30] They asked recently discharged patients to help them develop interventions to improve patient care. A discharge teaching package was designed and distributed to every unit in the hospital. On re-surveying patients one year after implementation they found statistically significant decreases in the frequency of problems related to discharge and an overall improvement in the continuity and transition dimension of the survey. Similar initiatives using systematic patient feedback to stimulate quality improvements have been reported from a number of hospitals in the US and Europe.

The survey results show that patients want to be confident that their doctors are acting in their best interests, but nurses also play a very important role in ensuring the quality of patient care. Nurses who are enthusiastic about patient feedback can make an important difference. For example, a nurse-led unit in the University Hospital of Umeå in Sweden commissioned a patient survey in 1997 and used the results to initiate change in three key areas: admission routines, ward organisation, and pain relief.[31] In the 1997 survey 29% of patients with pre-booked admissions reported a long wait before they were allocated a bed. Staff discussed the problem and decided to reorganise the admissions process. When a second survey was carried out in 2000, the proportion of patients reporting long waits was down to 14%. Similar improvements were achieved in the proportion of patients who said there were insufficient opportunities to talk to a nurse when necessary – down from 19% to 10% following staff training and reorganisation into smaller work groups – and in pain relief, where the proportion of patients reporting a problem was reduced from 15% to 6% following retraining, reorganisation and provision of self-medication facilities.

Feedback to individual clinicians
Although many clinicians are given the results of patient surveys, little is known about how commonly this is done, how formalized the processes used are, and what is the impact on behaviour. Recently patient feedback has been introduced

into some general practice vocational training schemes. Using a patient questionnaire designed to provide feedback on interpersonal skills, doctors and nurses can be provided with patients' evaluation of their performance in relation to such things as the warmth of their greeting; their listening and explaining skills; the extent of reassurance provided to the patient; the patient's confidence in their ability; the opportunity they gave to the patient to express their concerns and fears; the respect shown to the patient and the time allocated for the consultation; their consideration of the patient's personal situation in treatment offered or advice given; their concern for the patient as a person; whether or not the patient would recommend them to their friends; and the patient's overall satisfaction with the consultation.

A patient feedback questionnaire covering the topics listed above was used with a group of doctors and nurses working in two district general hospitals in Devon.[32] Nurses achieved the best overall scores. Consultants scored highest in areas of 'respect shown to patient' and 'patients' confidence in their ability', and lowest in 'time given for visit'. Physicians scored significantly better than surgeons, but consultants scored significantly higher overall than junior doctors. An evaluation of this approach to obtaining and using patient feedback with Australian GP registrars found that it led to significant improvements in specific aspects such as listening skills, ability to elicit concerns and fears, time given to patients and the provision of reassurance.[33]

The GMC is now developing plans to use this type of direct feedback from patients in the revalidation process which all doctors will have to undergo every five years. Many doctors will find this procedure somewhat threatening. The published studies reflect the views of enthusiasts and may not be a good guide to what will happen when patient feedback becomes compulsory. However, if the results are used in a developmental rather than a punitive manner, in theory at least it could make a real difference to patients' experience. In spite of the intuitive appeal of this approach, simply feeding back data to clinicians has not resulted in the consistent and high levels of quality we would hope for.[34] There are several reports in the literature of positive benefits arising from feedback of patient survey data, but little systematic evidence that provider feedback on its own, without additional incentives to use the information to make changes, will be sufficient to stimulate large-scale quality improvements.[16;35] The trend now is towards a more systematic approach to incorporating patients', users' and carers' views into quality assessment with the results of such studies being incorporated into accreditation programmes and performance monitoring by external bodies.

Obtaining a national picture

In England all hospitals and primary care Trusts are now required to perform their own local patient surveys on an annual basis, including a standard set of questions for use in national performance monitoring and benchmarking. The first wave of acute Trust surveys were under way as I was preparing this monograph and the others will follow shortly. The hope is that Trusts will use the findings from these regular surveys to initiate quality improvements and monitor progress, but the requirements of top-down performance assessment and bottom-up quality improvement are hard to reconcile. National surveys can be implemented centrally and the results fed back to providers. In this way methodological quality can be assured and consistency in data analysis ensures that performance indicators derived from the surveys are valid and comparable. However, there may be no local 'ownership' of an externally-imposed survey and hence less inclination to act on the findings. National surveys also take a long time to organise, with resulting loss in timeliness of the results. Local surveys can be carried out much more quickly and providers are more likely to 'own' the results, but methodology and data quality may be inconsistent, giving potentially misleading results if they are used to make comparisons between different institutions.

To counter these problems the Department of Health has decided to coordinate a series of locally implemented surveys. Each Trust is required to organise and pay for their own patient survey using a standard 'core' set of questions, but they can add their own additional questions if they wish. The surveys have to be carried out according to a set of pre-determined methodological standards and the results must be submitted to the Department of Health for use in the national Performance Assessment Framework. It is hoped that these centrally coordinated, locally implemented surveys will achieve both goals: 'bottom-up' quality improvement and 'top-down' national monitoring of performance.

The initiatives announced in the NHS Plan mark a new departure for the health service in England. The government plans to use direct financial incentives for hospitals to stimulate quality improvements and data from national patient surveys are now included in the performance-related incentive scheme.[36] Results of the surveys will be published in the hope that this will encourage providers to ensure that their services are truly patient-centred. The plan places patients firmly at the centre of the government's attempt to modernise the health service and, as such, constitutes the first really concerted attempt to align a number of incentives – provider feedback, public disclosure, and financial incentives – to improve patients' experience.

These new incentive systems, coupled with the determination to increase NHS funding to match levels in other European countries, offer a real opportunity for improvement. If the roll out of these new policy initiatives is rigorously evaluated, they will also offer an unprecedented opportunity to learn more about the mechanisms for achieving system-wide change and the problems that have to be overcome if health care systems are to work really well for patients.

'Hard-to-reach' groups

Self-completion postal surveys are a useful way of gathering information from large populations relatively cheaply and they can be very helpful in pinpointing problems in specific minority groups. For example, the national surveys of general practice patients and patients with coronary heart disease revealed that people from minority ethnic groups, particularly those of Asian origin, reported more problems than people from the indigenous white population.[27;37] However, self-completion questionnaires have important limitations when seeking the views of people who speak minority languages, or those who have literacy problems, or particular disabilities, for example blindness or learning disabilities. People who are homeless or who move frequently, for example travellers and some people with mental illness, may also be excluded if postal surveys are the only method used. For these groups one needs to look to alternative methods of gaining feedback on patients' and families' experiences. Strategies can include qualitative techniques, such as in-depth interviews or focus groups, and special consultation exercises, including public meetings or participative research techniques organised in conjunction with community or user groups.

The value of undertaking specific exercises to target people from minority groups has been shown in many studies. For example, the beliefs and self-management strategies of many Asian patients with asthma were found to be misunderstood by their doctors, leading to poor communication, ineffective advice and inappropriate treatment decisions.[38] In one disadvantaged urban area in the UK, volunteers from the South Asian community were trained to carry out research among members of their own community.[39] This yielded important insights into psychological distress experienced by members of this disadvantaged group and led to various recommendations for improving health services in the area. The views of mental health patients and user groups in three areas of London were sought as part of a programme to improve the quality of primary health care for this group.[40] This study pinpointed the need for improvements in information about mental health problems, communication between health professionals and coordination of care, greater sensitivity and a better reception from staff in the clinic, longer consultation time, access to a wider range of health professionals, and less labelling and stigmatisation of mental health problems.

Performance indicators

The high cost of health care has led to pressure for greater public accountability, resulting in the publication of performance indicators designed to enable comparison between health care facilities. Public access to data on quality of care among different providers has developed much further in the USA than in the UK, but hospital report cards and physician profiles are now being promoted widely and the new emphasis on internet information is boosting these efforts. Recent developments among commercial websites, such as 'Dr Foster' (www.drfoster.co.uk), are encouraging patients to seek and use systematic information on health care quality.[41] The establishment in the UK of new mechanisms for promoting involvement and choice, including the establishment of Patient Forums and the requirement to publish a Patient Prospectus for each hospital and primary care Trust, will add a further boost to these efforts.[36]

The premises underlying the moves towards public disclosure of information on quality are that patients will use the information to select high quality providers and the selection process will motivate providers to improve the quality of care.[42] For this approach to work, the information provided must be perceived to be valid, salient to patients, presented in a useful, readable and accessible format, must influence, or be perceived to influence people's choice of provider, and providers with poor quality must fail and/or improve in response to this process.[43] Patients must also be persuaded that choice of provider is both feasible and desirable.

NHS Trust performance ratings may be useful for accountability purposes and for prompting investigations into the causes of variations in quality and outcome, but for the individual patient facing a decision about whether to go to a particular hospital for a specific treatment, general information about the quality of care aggregated across a whole Trust is unlikely to be much use. Instead this hypothetical patient is more likely to want information about the performance of the particular hospital specialty or department in which they are to be treated, or that of the specialist or team who will be responsible for their care. Even more useful would be success rates for the particular treatment or procedure they will undergo, with comparative information about alternative treatments or the same treatment performed by different teams if they face a choice. In its current form the NHS Performance Assessment Framework could provide some relevant information, for example waiting times for breast cancer treatment, mortality rates for hip fracture, stroke and coronary artery bypass grafts, but this type of information is limited to a few indicators and is difficult to find.[44]

Evidence on what type of information British patients want, if any, and what they might use it for, is sparse. Needless to say, this issue has been studied much more extensively in the USA, particularly in relation to choice of health plan. For example, qualitative research revealed that American patients wanted an unbiased, expert source of judgment about health care quality and they wanted to know how others "like them" evaluated care.[16] Interpersonal relations are a key factor in patients' evaluations of health plans. A national survey of American healthcare consumers' information needs found that the quality of doctors was considered the most important factor in choosing a health plan, followed by courtesy and manner of the physicians and staff, the ability to choose one's own doctors, specialists and hospital, and the cost of the plan.[45]

Information on process and outcome indicators in different hospitals has been a feature of the American scene for some years. Despite the fact that these indicators reveal considerable variations in performance between hospitals, very few patients are aware of the data and even fewer seem to use it.[46] A number of explanations have been proposed to account for American consumers' failure to use the published indicators. These include the following:

1. Consumers are not aware of variations in quality so don't seek information about 'the best' providers.[47]

2. Consumers don't believe they have a choice or prefer to leave it to their employer to choose a plan.[48]
3. Relevant information is not available at the time it is needed.[46]
4. Healthcare report cards are badly designed and consumers find them hard to understand.[49-51]
5. Consumers don't trust the information or its source.[47]

Despite the lack of evidence that report cards are being used by American consumers, there is still a considerable commitment to the principle of public disclosure of information about healthcare quality.[52;53] Those consumers who are aware of the report cards say they find them helpful and relevant even if they use them only rarely. Public disclosure of healthcare performance information is still at an early stage in the diffusion curve even in the USA. We need to wait a few years before the full impact can be properly assessed.

In the meantime, the British government is committed to making information available to the public, both via the official publication of performance indicators and by supplying information to commercial providers such as Dr. Foster. While Americans are used to the idea that market competition is an inevitable feature of healthcare, this notion is more foreign to the British public. The British government wants to encourage patients to exercise choice and behave more like consumers, but choice is less celebrated here and accountability of public services to the taxpayers who fund them may provide a stronger motivation for British people to take notice of the data.

A key issue will be whether greater transparency enhances or undermines public confidence in the NHS.[54;55] In a recent series of BBC Reith lectures, the philosopher Oonora O'Neil questioned the basis for the new emphasis on performance measurement as a tool for accountability, arguing that it distorts the proper aims of professional practice and imposes inconsistent forms of central control.[56] Trust in public services does not seem to have been strengthened by the plethora of indicators:

"In the very years in which the accountability revolution has made striking advances, in which increased demands for control and performance, scrutiny and audit have been imposed, and in which the performance of professionals and institutions has been more and more controlled, we find in fact growing reports of mistrust."[56]

Of course British patients do have to make choices, for example about which general practice or dentist to register with when they move into a new area, or whether to accept a recommendation for referral or treatment, or to opt out of the NHS and seek private healthcare. The evidence suggests that personal recommendation is the major influence on choice of primary care provider and waiting time is still the dominant concern when making choices related to secondary care.[57] However, other issues feature strongly as well; for example, well-trained staff, up-to-date treatment and hygienic wards were rated highly in a Consumers' Association survey.[58] A survey conducted by MORI on behalf of the Audit Commission revealed high levels of ignorance about how the NHS is performing or how to find information to assist in choosing a provider.[59] About half of those surveyed said they would be interested in receiving comparative information about health services and NHS performance and there was considerable interest in obtaining this information via GPs, although there was also a demand for it to be available from a variety of sources.

A recent study involving 50 patients and members of the public in six focus groups organised around England looked at patients' and public views of performance indicators.[60] There was general agreement that some form of monitoring of NHS facilities was a good idea, but people were ambivalent about the value of the current set of indicators. Participants wanted information about specific local services that they could relate to their particular situation rather than generalised comparative information. They thought this information should be publicly available, but they felt they had little choice about where they were treated so the information would be of limited use. Even if choice were possible, most participants did not like the idea of "shopping around" for health care and expected a high standard of care everywhere. Although there was recognition that the publication of performance information might encourage improvement in performance, there was also widespread concern that it would demoralise an already demoralised workforce and make staff retention even more difficult.

Publication of information about the quality and performance of health care has had only limited effect to date but there are signs that patients are becoming more sophisticated as consumers of health services and are increasingly willing to travel to secure the 'best' quality.[47;61] Measures of patient experience may prove easier for patients to interpret than other measures of performance such as mortality rates. Awareness that these data are publicly available may prove to be an effective incentive for providers to ensure that their services are truly patient-centred.

REFERENCES

[1] Delbanco T, Berwick DM, Boufford J, Edgman-Levitan S et al. Healthcare in a land caled PeoplePower: nothing about me without me. Health Expectations 2001; **4**: 144–150.

[2] Birch Q, Field S, Scrivens E. Quality in general practice. Abingdon: Radcliffe Medical Press, 2000.

[3] Bruster, S., Lilley, S-J., Lorentzon, M., and Richards, N. Focus groups report. 1999. Edinburgh, Lothian University Hospitals NHS Trust.

[4] Grol R, Wensing M, Mainz J, Jung HP, Ferreira P, Hearnshaw H *et al*. Patients in Europe evaluate general practice care: an international comparison. *British Journal of General Practice* 2000;50:882–7.

[5] Carr-Hill RA. The measurement of patient satisfaction. *Journal of Public Health Medicine* 1992;**14**:236–49.

[6] Hall JA,.Dornan MC. What patients like about their medical care and how often they are asked: a meta-analysis of the satisfaction literature. *Social Science and Medicine* 1988;**27**:935–9.

[7] Sitzia J,.Wood N. Patient satisfaction: a review of issues and concepts. *Social Science and Medicine* 1998;**45**:1829–43.

[8] Fitzpatrick R,.Hopkins A. Problems in the conceptual framework of patient satisfaction research: an empirical exploration. *Sociology of Health and Illness* 2000;**5**:297–311.

[9] Edwards C,.Staniszewska S. Accessing the user's perspective. *Health and Social Care in the Community* 2000;**8**:417–24.

[10] Cleary PD. The increasing importance of patient surveys. *British Medical Journal* 1999;**319**:720–1.

[11] Cleary PD,.Edgman-Levitan S. Health care quality: incorporating consumer perspectives. *Journal of the American Medical Association* 1997;**278**:1608–12.

[12] Cleary PD, Edgman-Levitan S, Walker JD, Gerteis M, Delbanco TD. Using patient reports to improve medical care: a preliminary report from 10 hospitals. *Quality Management in Health Care* 1993;**2**:31–8.

[13] Beatrice DF, Thomas CP, Biles B. Grant making with an impact: the Picker/Commonwealth patient-centred care program. *Health Affairs* 1998;**17**:236–44.

[14] Edgman-Levitan S,.Cleary PD. What information do consumers want and need? *Health Affairs* 1996;**15**:42–56.

[15] Gerteis M, Edgman-Levitan S, Daley J, Delbanco TL. Through the patient's eyes: understanding and promoting patient-centred care. San Francisco: Jossey Bass, 1993.

[16] Cleary PD, Edgman-Levitan S, Roberts M, Moloney TW, McMullen W, Walker JD *et al.* Patients evaluate their hospital care: a national survey. *Health Affairs* 1991;**10**:254–67.

[17] Delbanco TL, Stokes DM, Cleary PD, Edgman-Levitan S, Walker JD, Gerteis M *et al.* Medical patients' assessments of their care during hospitalization. *Journal of General Internal Medicine* 1995;**10**:679–85.

[18] Draper M, Cohen P, Buchan H. Seeking consumer views: what use are results of hospital patient satisfaction surveys? *International Journal for Quality in Health Care* 2001;**13**:463–8.

[19] Charles C, Gauld M, Chambers L, O'Brien B, Haynes R, Labelle R. How was your hospital stay? Patients' reports about their care in Canadian hospitals. *Canadian Medical Association Journal* 1994;**150**:1813–22.

[20] Bruster S, Jarman B, Bosanquet N, Weston D, Erens R, Delbanco TL. National survey of hospital patients. *British Medical Journal* 1994;**309**:1542–6.

[21] Coulter A,.Cleary PD. Patients' experiences with hospital care in five countries. *Health Affairs* 2001;**20**:244–52.

[22] Gulacsi L. Quality of hospital care: patient satisfaction and patients reports in Hungarian hospitals, 1992–1997. In Gulasci L, ed. *Hungarian Health Care in Transition*, pp 147–84. University of Amsterdam: Department of Social Medicine, 2001.

[23] Bechel DL, Myers WA, Smith DG. Does patient-centred care pay off? *Journal on Quality Improvement* 2000;**26**:400–9.

[24] Fremont AM, Cleary PD, Hargraves JL, Rowe RM, Jacobson NB, Ayanian JZ. Patient-centred processes of care and long-term outcomes of myocardial infarction. *Journal of General Internal Medicine* 2001;**16**:800–8.

[25] Murray CJL, Kawabata K, Valentine N. People's experience versus people's expectations. *Health Affairs* 2001;**20**:21–4.

[26] Carman KL, Short PF, Farley DO, Schnaier JA, Elliott DB, Gallagher PM. Early lessons from CAHPS demonstrations and evaluations. *Medical Care* 1999;**37**:MS97–MS105.

[27] Airey, C., Bruster, S., Calderwood, L., Erens, B., Pitson, L., Prior, G., and Richards, N. National survey of NHS patients: coronary heart disease 1999. Summary of key findings. 2001. London, Department of Health.

[28] Ovretveit J. Comparative and cross-cultural health research. Abingdon: Radcliffe Medical Press, 1998.

[29] Grol R, Wensing M, Mainz J, Ferreira P, Hearnshaw H, Hjortdahl P *et al.* Patients' priorities with respect to general practice care: an international comparison. *Family Practice* 1999;16: 4–11.

[30] Reiley P, Pike A, Phipps M, Weiner M, Miller N, Stengrevics S *et al.* Learning from patients: a discharge planning improvement project. *Quality Improvement* 1996;22:311–22.

[31] Frantzen, K. and Hoglund, E. Learn from your patients! European Forum for Quality in Health Care conference, Bologna (poster) . 2001.

[32] Greco M, Sweeney K, Broomhall J, Beasley P. Patient assessment of interpersonal skills: a clinical governance activity for hospital doctors and nurses. *Journal of Clinical Excellence* 2001;3:117–24.

33 Greco M, Brownlea A, McGovern J. Impact of patient feedback on the interpersonal skills of general practice registrars: results of a longtudinal study. Medical Education 2001;35:748–56.

34 Schuster MA, McGlynn EA, Brook RH. How good is quality of health care in the United States? *Milbank Quarterly* 1998;76:517–63.

35 Wedderburn Tate C, Bruster S, Broadley K, Maxwell E, Stevens L. What do patients really think? *Health Services Journal* 1995;12th January:18–20.

36 Secretary of State for Health. The NHS Plan: a plan for investment, a plan for reform. 2000. London, Stationery Office.

37 Department of Health. National survey of NHS patients: general practice 1998. Airey, C. and Erens, B. 2002. London, Department of Health.

38 Lomax H, Brooks F, Mitchell M. Understanding user health care strategies: experiences of asthma therapy among South Asians and White cultural groups. In Gillam S, Brooks F, eds. *New Beginnings: Towards patient and public involvement in primary health care*, pp 77–89. London: King's Fund, 2001.

39 Kai J,.Hedges C. Minority ethnic community participation in needs assessment and service development in primary care: perceptions of Pakistani and Bangladeshi people about psychological distress. *Health Expectations* 1999;2:7–20.

40 Greatley, A. and Peck, E. Mental health priorities for primary care. 1999. London, King's Fund.

41 Dr Foster. www.drfoster.co.uk . 2002.

42 Marshall MN. Accountability and quality improvement: the role of report cards. *Quality in Health Care* 2001;10:68.

43 Draper, M. and Hill, S. The role of patient satisfaction surveys in a national approach to hospital quality management. 1995. Canberra, Australian Government Publishing Service.

44 Department of Health. NHS Performance Indicators: National Summary. February. 2002.

45 Isaacs SL. Consumers' information needs: results of a national survey. *Health Affairs* 1996;15:31–41.

46 Schneider EC,.Epstein AM. Use of public performance reports: a survey of patients undergoing cardiac surgery. *Journal of the American Medical Association* 1998;279:1638–42.

47 Schneider EC,.Lieberman T. Publicly disclosed information about the quality of health care: response of the US public. *Quality in Health Care* 2001;10:96–103.

48 Hoy EW, Wicks EK, Forland RA. A guide to facilitating consumer choice. *Health Affairs* 1996;15:9–30.

49 Hibbard JH, Slovic P, Peters E, Finucane ML, Tusler M. Is the informed-choice policy approach appropriate for Medicare beneficiaries? *Health Affairs* 2001;20:199–203.

50 Veroff DR, Gallagher PM, Wilson V, Uyeda M, Merselis J, Guadagnoli E et al. Effective reports for health care quality data: lessons from a CAHPS demonstration in Washington State. *International Journal of Quality in Health Care* 1998;10:555–60.

51 Vaiana ME,.McGlynn EA. What cognitive science tells us about the design of reports for consumers. *Medical Care Research and Review* 2002;59:3–35.

[52] Clancy CM. Consumer preferences: path to improvement? *Health Services Research* 1999;34:807–11.

[53] Hibbard JH, Berkman N, Jael E. The impact of a CAHPS report on employee knowledge, beliefs and decisions. *Medical Care Research and Review* 2002;59:104–16.

[54] Brownlea A. Earning confidence: perspectives for a modernising NHS. *Journal of Clinical Excellence* 2001;3:27–32.

[55] Mulligan J. What do the public think? *Health Care UK* 2000;Winter:12–7.

[56] O'Neil, O. Lecture 3: Called to account. Reith lectures. www.bbc.co.uk/radio4 . 2002. BBC.

[57] Higgins J,.Wiles R. Study of patients who chose private health care for treatment. *British Journal of General Practice* 2001;42:326–9.

[58] Consumers' Association. What consumers want from the NHS. brief report 2001.

[59] MORI for Audit Commission. Local commentaries on NHS health services. 2001.

[60] Magee, H., Coulter, A., and Davis, L. J. Patient and public views on performance indicators: a focus group study. 2002. Oxford, Picker Institute Europe.

[61] Marshall MN, Shekelle PG, Leatherman S, Brook RH. The public release of performance data: What do we expect to gain? A review of the evidence. *Journal of the American Medical Association* 2000;283:1866–74.

[62] Coulter A, Cleary P. Measuring and improving patients' experiences: how can we make health care systems work for patients? Measuring up: improving health systems performance in OECD countries, pp 211–24. Paris: OECD, 2002.

6. Rights, responsibilities and accountability: patient as active citizen

"The citizen's voice and choice should make as significant a contribution to shaping health care services as the decisions taken at other levels of economic, managerial and professional decision-making."[1]

WHO, Ljubljana Charter on Reforming Health Care, 1996

A role for the citizen?

As citizens all patients have rights, but until recently these rights were mostly laid down in professional codes of practice which were not well understood by lay people. It was not felt to be necessary to inform people of their rights. The assumption was that the bodies concerned with professional self-regulation would ensure that patients were protected and if any health professionals failed to abide by their codes of conduct, they had their own mechanisms for dealing with them. The legal system provided a back-up in cases of very serious breaches.

The steep rise in litigation rates was the most obvious sign that self-regulation was not perceived to be providing sufficient protection for patients. However, it is still the case that only a small minority of patients resort to the law when something goes wrong. Dissatisfied patients have other options, including making a formal complaint, and, if this does not produce an acceptable response, taking the issue to an Ombudsman. But these systems for seeking redress were a necessary but insufficient response to the new desire for more accountability. What was felt to be needed was a stronger role for patients in the regulatory bodies and more public involvement in the development of health policy. In their *Declaration on the promotion of patients' rights in Europe*, WHO outlined various strategies which could be adopted to strengthen involvement at each of the three policy levels – clinical, local, and national.[2] These included clarifying patients' rights and entitlements, for example by issuing patients' charters, strengthening the voice of the user by supporting patient groups, and improving public information about health care to stimulate constructive debate about priorities.

Patients' charters

Patients' rights legislation was a phenomenon of the nineties. Throughout the decade many countries introduced patients rights laws or patients charters to clarify these rights.[3] That this legislation was considered necessary was an interesting reflection on changing attitudes to health care – a sign that people had become less willing to trust health professionals to safeguard their rights. Patients' rights legislation in these countries covered all or some of the following topics: the right to confidentiality, to information and informed consent, to refuse or halt treatment, to choose a health care provider, to have access to medical records, to be free of discrimination, to respect and dignity and to self-determination. Patients' charters were intended as a means of drawing attention to patients' rights, thereby strengthening them and setting down standards which could be publicly monitored.

The UK Patient's Charter was introduced in 1992. It set out ten 'rights' to which every patient was entitled (Box 1):

Box 1

UK patients' rights[4]

- To receive health care on the basis of clinical need, regardless of ability to pay
- To be registered with a GP
- To receive emergency medical care at any time, through your GP or the emergency ambulance service and hospital accident and emergency departments
- To be referred to a consultant, acceptable to you, when your GP thinks it necessary, and to be referred for a second opinion if you and your GP agree this is desirable
- To be given a clear explanation of any treatment proposed, including any risks and any alternatives, before you decide whether you will agree to the treatment
- To have access to your health records, and to know that those working for the NHS are under a legal duty to keep their contents confidential

- To choose whether or not you wish to take part in medical research or medical student training
- To be given detailed information on local health services, including quality standards and maximum waiting times
- To be guaranteed admission for treatment by a specific date no later than two years from the day when your consultant places you on a waiting list
- To have any complaint about NHS services – whoever provides them – investigated and to receive a full and prompt written reply from the chief executive or general manager.

Patient's Charter, 1992

While helpful in the sense of raising awareness and setting standards, the legislation did not necessarily advance patients' legal rights as much as it might have appeared. Although the Patient's Charter used the language of rights, most of these took the form of general statutory duties rather than legally enforceable individual entitlements. The first seven of the rights in the Patient's Charter were simply restatements of existing legislation. The last three were new commitments on minimum waiting times and response to complaints. These were later amended to accommodate revised commitments to shorter minimum waiting times. They were accompanied by a list of national and local standards against which performance would be measured. These included waiting times for ambulance services, for initial assessment in accident and emergency services and in outpatient clinics, cancellation of operations, and arrangements for hospital discharge.

The Patients' Charter was introduced by a Conservative government. When they came to power in 1997 the new Labour government commissioned a review of the Patients' Charter. This was critical of the way it had been implemented and of its unintended consequences.[5;6] Many NHS staff resented the fact that the charter had been imposed on them by the government. They had not been consulted about its development and were therefore not fully committed to achieving the goals it set. They saw it as a stick for the government to beat them with and they felt it led to a distortion of priorities. The standards focused on access, largely because waiting times were easily measurable. Staff felt under pressure to give higher priority to patients with minor problems over those with more serious clinical needs, just to avoid looking bad in the waiting list statistics.

The emphasis on league tables and competition encouraged providers to cheat to make their statistics look good. For example, many accident and emergency departments introduced so-called 'hello' nurses to greet patients within the five minutes laid down by the Charter standard, but they were then left to wait long hours before their needs were attended to. Staff also felt the Charter encouraged patients to have unrealistic expectations, and to complain, without placing any obligations or responsibilities on them.

Most patients had heard about the Charter but were very unclear about its contents and its intentions. There was a mismatch between patients' concerns and Charter priorities. Patients wanted more information about treatment options, and they were interested in primary as well as secondary care, which was barely covered by the charter standards. Although the Charter promised patients the right to full information and the opportunity to participate in decisions about their care, the reality for most patients fell far short of the aspiration. Since there was no measurable standard for this aspect of the Charter, it was not seen as a priority.

Following this review, the government promised to replace the Patients' Charter with a new charter which would emphasise patients' responsibilities as well as their rights and would include a guide for the public on how to access health services. When it finally appeared, *Your Guide to the NHS* looked very different from the *Patient's Charter*.[7] All mention of "rights" had been expunged, to be replaced by "commitments", "responsibilities" and "expectations". The new approach was intended to look more like a contract between the NHS and its users than a charter. It set out a range of commitments and responsibilities on both sides (Table 1):

It is hard to object to any of the specific sentiments expressed, but the tone of the Guide is very different from the Charter that it replaced. It seems more designed to reassure staff than to empower patients and it smacks strongly of a return to paternalism. Gone are the commitments to information and choice. Instead we are exhorted to look after ourselves and not to bother professionals unnecessarily. It seems unlikely that the Guide will have much impact unless it is accompanied by incentives for staff and patients to use it and a mechanism for monitoring any deviations from the 'contract'. To date it is unclear what, if anything, the government intends to do about this.

TABLE 1

Commitments and responsibilities in *Your Guide to the NHS*

NHS commitments	*Patients' responsibilities*
The NHS will provide a universal service for all based on clinical need, not ability to pay.	Do what you can to look after your own health and follow advice on a healthy lifestyle.
The NHS will provide a comprehensive range of services.	Care for yourself when appropriate. (For example you can treat yourself at home for common ailments such as coughs, colds and sore throats.)
The NHS will shape its services around the needs and preferences of individual patients, their families and carers.	Give blood if you are able, and carry an organ donor card or special needs card or bracelet.
The NHS will respond to different needs of different populations.	Listen carefully to advice on your treatment and medication. Tell the doctor about any treatments you are already taking.
The NHS will work continuously to improve quality services and to minimise errors.	Treat NHS staff, fellow patients, carers and visitors politely, and with respect. We will not accept violence, racial, sexual or verbal harassment.
The NHS will support and value its staff.	Keep your appointment or let the GP, dentist, clinic or hospital know as soon as possible if you cannot make it. Book routine appointments in plenty of time.
Public funds for healthcare will be devoted solely to NHS patients.	Return any equipment that is no longer needed.
The NHS will keep people healthy and work to reduce health inequalities.	Pay NHS prescription charges and any other charges promptly when they are due and claim financial benefits or exemptions from these charges correctly.
The NHS will respect the confidentiality of individual patients and provide open access to information about services, treatment and performance.	Use this Guide to help you find the services you need.

Direct participation

In most of the countries where they were introduced, patients' charters avoided any definition of the scope of coverage or the amount of resources to be devoted to health care. The focus on the rights of the individual patient tended to divert attention from the need to strengthen democratic control of health systems and to foster citizen's empowerment in a political sense. [8;9] Charters can be useful for setting standards and focusing attention on certain rights, but they need to be supplemented by other strategies to increase participation.

The WHO declaration on patients' rights emphasised the importance of strong patient groups and called upon governments to support them financially. Some countries, for example the Netherlands, have an extensive network of patient groups which attract government funding and high levels of participation. The UK also has a large number of voluntary patient groups, most of which receive no government funds. It also has a long tradition of statutory groups established with government funding.

Twenty five years ago the British government made a limited, but nevertheless important, direct investment in user groups when it established the Community Health Councils (CHCs). These were introduced in 1974 to represent user interests at local level. Each CHC had eighteen members appointed by the health authority, the local councils and the voluntary sector. Wholly funded by the Department of Health, albeit not very generously, they were independent of local providers and health authorities. They were expected to represent the public interest in the work of these bodies and they had a statutory right to be consulted about major plans and a legal duty to monitor services by inspecting premises, reviewing performance against Patient's Charter standards and assisting complainants. Beyond this their role was never very clear. CHCs engaged in a wide variety of activities, ranging from advocacy on behalf of individual patients, or preparing detailed comments on local plans, to working with local agencies to promote public health.

During their 25 year existence some CHCs succeeded in making considerable impact at local level, but others were less successful. [10-13] Lacking formal procedures for election to their Boards, they tended to be unrepresentative bodies dependent on the energy and commitment of unpaid volunteers (often with a specific vested interest) and a very small number of paid staff. To some extent their role was eroded by successive waves of policy innovation in which, for example, health authorities were given lead responsibility for public consultation and hospitals and health authorities established better systems for dealing with complaints. The recent establishment of the Commission for Health Improvement further undermined their role. The CHCs felt left alone, like Cinderella, exploited and unloved while the party moved on elsewhere. Then the government decided to kill them off and delegate their functions to a raft of new bodies, including the Patient Advice and Liaison Service (PALS), the Independent Complaints Advisory Service (ICAS), Patients' Forums in each Trust, and the Commission for Patient and Public Involvement in Health.[14;15]

The decision to abolish the CHCs was the most controversial of all the proposals outlined in the NHS Plan. Ironically it galvanised the CHCs into an unprecedented frenzy of lobbying activity which attracted considerable political support. At the time of writing (May 2002) the NHS Reform and Health Care Professions Bill is still the subject of fierce debate, and looks unlikely to get through both Houses of Parliament unscathed. Campaigners have been trying to ensure that CHCs are replaced by independent patients' councils which would have wider powers and stronger teeth than the Patients' Forums favoured by the government. While it is undoubtedly true that the effectiveness of local CHCs was variable and there was real need for reform of their remit, funding and governance arrangements, abolishing them and replacing them with non-independent bodies looks like a retrograde step, and possibly an expensive mistake.

Voluntary patient organisations

The majority of patient organisations are 'single issue' groups. Single issue groups include those which organise around a particular disease or clinical problem, for example, the Multiple Sclerosis Society or Diabetes Care, and those which deal with a specific population group, for example the National Childbirth Trust or the Afro-Caribbean Mental Health Association. Some of these organisations are large and professionally-run, while others are small self-help groups operating with limited funds. Their functions include campaigning and lobbying, fundraising for research and service provision, advice and self-help. Some of the larger groups combine all these functions.

The plethora of groups has spawned some umbrella bodies, such as the Long-Term Medical Conditions Alliance which brings together about 60 organisations to promote the interests of more than a million people with chronic illness. There are also some generic patient associations which concern themselves with issues common to all patients, not just those with particular diseases. The single issue groups generally find it easier to attract committed participants than do the generic groups. For example, the Patient's Association, a relatively high profile national group, faced funding difficulties for some years. With no obvious constituency of people with long-term needs and therefore a long-term interest in its work, it cannot rely on a large membership for financial support so is forced to turn to government, charitable or commercial sources for funding.

The pharmaceutical industry has shown considerable interest in funding patient groups, particularly those groups campaigning on behalf of patients who might be persuaded to consume their products. Direct-to-consumer advertising is currently prohibited within the European Union but organisations like the Association of British Pharmaceutical Industries have aimed to foster close relations with patient groups as a key plank of their public relations strategy. Some patient groups were established with funding from pharmaceutical companies as part of their 'disease awareness' campaigns, while others were set up by clinicians to support their efforts to raise funds for research. Although many reputable groups are scrupulous about avoiding any strings that might be attached to industry funding, not all are so fastidious. Some so-called 'patient groups' are vehicles for industry public relations rather than genuine user groups. The representativeness of many of these groups is therefore open to doubt.

Concerns about representativeness have also been voiced about patient participation groups in general practice. These groups have a fairly long history dating back to the 1970s when the National Association for Patient Participation was founded.[16] The majority of these groups were in rural or small town areas and were usually associated with larger group practices. Most were initiated by GPs and they engaged in a variety of activities including the provision of services (for example, transport and prescription collection schemes, visiting and befriending, running crèches and fundraising), providing feedback about practice organization (including suggestion boxes, surveys and open meetings), and health promotion or community development (including lectures, discussion groups, self-help groups and campaigning on local issues). However, few groups managed to persuade large numbers of patients to get involved and those that did tended to be 'the usual suspects', i.e. middle class, middle aged women.[17]

A two-year study of patients' associations in Britain and America concluded that despite their potential collective strength as multi-million pound (or dollar) charities with large memberships and considerable numbers of paid employees, they had largely failed to exert themselves as a constructive political lobby on behalf of patients generally.[18] Many were concerned to increase and improve the services for the specific groups of patients they represented, but this was rarely accompanied by a radical critique of the system. Furthermore the fragmentation of groups mitigated against collective action. In some cases they had allowed themselves to be used as sources of manpower and funds to supplement basic services, tolerated by the government but not seen as a key player in policy-making. There were some honourable exceptions to this rule, however. For example groups concerned with HIV/AIDS developed into a highly effective lobby which has achieved much at national and international levels, people with mental health problems have a very effective champion in MIND, the National Association for Mental Health, and some of the umbrella groups, such as the Long-term Medical Conditions Alliance (LMCA), have also developed into professional and effective lobbies. Strong campaigns by the National Childbirth Trust (NCT) and the National Association for the Welfare of Children in Hospital (NAWCH) led to important changes in policy, and groups such as Diabetes UK and the Stroke Association have made substantial contributions to the development of national standards as embodied in the National Service Frameworks.

Patient groups now have an opportunity to play an even more influential role. The British government has announced its intention to "move away from a system of patients being on the outside, to one where the voices of patients, their carers and the public generally are heard and listened to through every level of the service, acting as a lever for change and improvement."[14] The plans include various mechanisms for increasing direct patient participation in oversight of provider performance, including the establishment of Patients' Forums in every acute and primary care Trust which are intended to be "truly representative of a broad sweep of the community."

There are still a number of hurdles to be overcome though. There may be difficulties in filling the 'lay' places on these committees. The dangers of tokenism in patient representation on committees are well recognised and the plans envisage a much greater number of lay representatives than ever before. Despite their potential collective strength, many individual patient groups are small, poorly funded, and dependent on volunteers. The relatively few umbrella or general groups cannot be expected to supply members for all the new committees. There are fears that the new Patient Forums will not be sufficiently independent from Trust management, that they may attract people with a particular axe to grind, and will not represent the views of disadvantaged members of local communities who are unlikely to put themselves forward for membership.

While welcoming the new commitment to user involvement, it is important to recognise the limitations of direct participation. Since most patients are not members of organised groups, these groups cannot be said to represent the views of the majority. While most patients want providers to take account of their views and experiences, only a small unrepresentative minority will want to be actively involved in committees to achieve this. It will be crucial to ensure that the Patients Forums have access to regular feedback from representative samples of patients and citizens to balance the views of the special interest groups. The new NHS survey programme should serve a useful purpose here. Patients Forums could monitor the conduct and results of these surveys and ensure that appropriate action is taken to address any problems identified.

Seeking the views of citizens

The Ljubljana Charter on reforming health care stressed the importance of listening to the citizen's voice and choice. Achieving this goal depends on the development of effective mechanisms for seeking the views of members of the public. Throughout the nineties the British government made various attempts to foster public engagement in health service policy-making. The *Local Voices* initiative was launched by the Department of Health in 1992.[19] Health authorities were urged to involve local people in their purchasing activities and to consult them about priorities for resource allocation. Some local health authorities embraced this duty with enthusiasm, while others gave it minimal effort. A wide variety of public consultation techniques were tried. Some used surveys, others distributed reports or leaflets outlining their plans, together with questionnaires designed to elicit the views of local people. Response rates as low as 25–30% were common and one authority received only 65 replies from a distribution of 122,000 leaflets![20]

Many health authorities organised public meetings to consult on their plans, while others used focus groups. Somerset Health Authority established a series of eight health panels, each comprised of twelve people selected using a purposive sampling technique to ensure that they were balanced in terms of age, sex and socio-economic group.[21] The groups, which met three times a year, had a rolling membership with four new people joining and four retiring at each panel meeting. The health authority chose the topics for discussion and provided panel members with information which they were encouraged to discuss with friends and family prior to the meeting. Panel members were reminded that resources were limited and after about half an hour's discussion they were asked to vote on whether or not the health authority should purchase the particular service or treatment.

In many ways the health panels resembled citizen's juries, which have also been the subject of enthusiastic experimentation by health authorities.[22;23] The main difference is that juries meet over a period of several days, during which time they have the opportunity to meet and question a number of expert witnesses. After considerable deliberation between the sixteen or so jurors, a report is produced for the health authority summarising their views and outlining their recommendations. Juries have tackled topics such as improving the quality of life for mental health service users, priorities for improving palliative care, shifting GP services to other members of the primary care team, location of gynaecological cancer services, and funding complementary therapies for back pain sufferers. Citizen's juries have shown themselves to be perfectly capable of absorbing complex information and making sensible recommendations, but setting up the juries is costly and time-consuming and, since no group of only sixteen people can possible represent the diversity of views in a population of about 300,000, they cannot be said to be representative. Variations on this technique, such as deliberative polls and future search conferences, can be used to involve much larger groups, but they are considerably more difficult and expensive to set up.

Primary care trusts (PCTs) are required to put in place mechanisms to encourage public involvement. This is but one of a long list of responsibilities they face as new organisations. The task has been interpreted in many different ways to date and most have found it quite difficult.[24] Some did little more than invite a few lay people to join their committees, others set up patients panels or community forums, appointed link workers, developed relationships with local voluntary organisations, commissioned research or engaged in various forms of community outreach. In all cases sustaining the activities depended on the commitment of a few key individuals and it was not easy. People were often unclear about what they hoped to achieve by involving the public and in many cases it was hard to see any impact resulting from all the efforts. Usually this aspect of the PCT's work was under-resourced and it sometimes felt 'grafted on' or marginalized instead of being a fundamental part of the organisational development. The tensions between institutional and lay agendas were never far from the surface. Nevertheless, there have been some successes and it would be unrealistic to hope that dramatic change would occur overnight. Most people struggling to engage the public in local primary care organisations remain committed to the process despite the difficulties. As the authors of the King's Fund report remarked:

> "Public involvement is a form of dialogue, of uncovering and valuing difference. This seems to us to be worthwhile, wherever it may lead."[24]

Determining priorities

Equitable access to health care on the basis of need, not ability to pay, is a key goal for most people concerned about health policy. The increasing gap between public expectations and the supply of services has led policy-makers to consider new ways to ensure that limited resources are used efficiently and equitably. In the past politicians were often reluctant to spell out for members of the public the financial consequences of their demands for health care. They preferred to propagate the idea that all demands could be met if only efficiency could be increased. This attitude is changing as it becomes clear that the potential for medical technologies to achieve beneficial effects for larger numbers of people with a wider range of conditions and ailments is increasing faster than the public's willingness to pay for them. Rationing has always been a feature of health care in every country, but payers and policy-makers – including governments, insurers and managed care organisations – have been reluctant to talk about it. Now at last there are signs that it is coming out of the closet.

The key issue for the future is how to ensure fair and equitable distribution of health care resources. Which essential services should be available free at the point of use or at low cost and which should not? This is a time of rapid innovation in medical science. Conditions that were previously considered untreatable can now be treated. The boundaries of health care are extending. Now we have effective treatments for erectile dysfunction, for slimming and even for baldness! Should these be available to all those who want them or should they be considered a luxury available only to those who are prepared to pay? These decisions should not be taken behind closed doors by finance officers. In a democratic society the public, or their elected representatives, should decide.

Decisions to restrict or ration services are not amenable to a technical fix. They can and should be informed by evidence on clinical effectiveness, but they also involve values. The views of experts should be weighed alongside the opinions and experience of lay people. The American philosopher, Norman Daniels, has argued that policy-makers should seek public legitimacy for rationing decisions by meeting four criteria for 'reasonableness'.[25] The rationale for decisions to restrict access should be: clearly and publicly stated; it should be contestable and be acceptable to 'fair minded' people; there should be a mechanism for appeal; and the process should be enforceable and defensible.

There has been intense media interest in cases where individual patients have been denied access to specific high-cost treatments such as interferon beta for multiple sclerosis, donepezil for Alzheimer's disease, or in-vitro fertilisation to treat infertility.[7] Denial of these treatments to patients on the basis of non-clinical criteria such as where they happen to live has been seen (correctly) as an example of rationing in action. Health authorities under pressure to meet budget targets have made different decisions about which expensive treatments they will pay for. Press stories about patients in neighbouring authorities apparently having different entitlements to treatment have proved shocking to a public accustomed to thinking about the NHS as a fair and equitable service.

The government established the National Institute of Clinical Excellence (NICE) to provide guidance to the NHS on clinical effectiveness, cost effectiveness and clinical audit methods. Its aim is to "produce clear guidance for clinicians about which treatments work best for which patients". Importantly they have recognised that this evidence-based guidance must be made available to non-clinicians as well. If clinical guidelines are to have an impact, they must be perceived as legitimate by patients and the public. That means that patient representatives should be involved in developing them, they should take account of evidence which is patient-centred, (i.e. reflects the patient's point of view on the relative importance of different health outcomes), the basis for the recommendations (including any value judgements) should be transparent, and they should allow scope for individual preferences in choosing between alternatives.

How much scope should be allowed for individual choice remains a matter for debate. In spite of concerns about equity, opinion can be easily swayed when special cases seem to demand special resources. The case of Jaymee Bowen (Child B), a ten year-old British girl suffering from leukaemia was a recent high profile example.[26] She was refused funding for a second bone marrow transplant. Her father's refusal to accept the recommendations of doctors and the health authority that further treatment was not in her best interests, attracted great public sympathy. The media likes to champion the individual versus the bureaucrats, even if the bureaucracy – in this case the health authority – has tried its best to represent the interests of the local population. It was easier to identify with the tragic case of one attractive ten year-old, than to empathise with the unknown people who might be denied treatment if Jaymee's care had been allowed to consume a considerable proportion of the health authority's resources.

Postcode prescribing arises when local health authorities or clinicians differ amongst themselves about which treatments they consider both affordable and appropriate to provide. This is the essence of rationing. When resources are limited the central question that has to be faced is: how should we choose which beneficial services should be offered to whom, and which should not? This begs a number of further questions. What is meant by 'beneficial' – how is benefit defined – and who is the 'we' who should do the choosing?

To answer the question about benefit you need two different types of information; evidence from well-conducted evaluations of the effects and costs of a treatment or service; and information about people's values and preferences, both the people who might use the service and the citizens who will pay for it. A beneficial service or intervention is one in which the benefits are seen to outweigh the risks and costs, in the eyes of the individual patient or service user and the wider public, as well as those of scientists, managers or health professionals. Postcode prescribing arises when purchasers in different parts of the country arrive at different answers in computing this cost-benefit equation, thus undermining the fundamental NHS value of equity or fairness.

NICE was set up in response to a belief that health care resources ought to be much more carefully targeted than they have been hitherto. Choosing between competing priorities has always been difficult. As the gap between public expectations and the availability of resources has grown ever wider, devolving decision-making responsibility to individual health authorities and clinicians has been a convenient way for national politicians to duck the issue. The change of tack was prompted by concern that public confidence in the NHS, and hence in the government itself, was in danger of seeping away. The government is taking this tentative step into the dangerous waters of explicit rationing because the political risk of *not* keeping the public informed about the choices that are being made on their behalf is beginning to look more dangerous than the traditional alternative of muddling through implicitly.

Some have argued that these attempts to promote participation are nothing more than window dressing, designed to disguise the absence of democratic accountability in the system. It is often stated that a centrally-run service like the NHS suffers from a 'democratic deficit' because it is not subject to formal control by locally elected representatives and cannot therefore be truly accountable to local people. There have been many calls to give responsibility for commissioning health services to locally elected councils. Others have argued against this proposition on the grounds that a centrally funded service requires accountability upwards to the Secretary of State, who is constitutionally responsible for the NHS and is accountable to Parliament. A move toward formal local democracy might create conflict and muddle and could lead to even greater inequities in service provision.[27] Meanwhile the national government shows no signs of wishing to cede power to local authorities. They retain at least a rhetorical commitment to citizen empowerment, encouraging local involvement while acting to strengthen the central mechanisms of accountability. Time will tell whether or not these goals are compatible.

REFERENCES

[1]   World Health Organisation. The Ljubljana Charter on reforming Health Care. 1996. Copenhagen, WHO Regional Office for Europe.

[2]   World Health Organisation. A declaration on the promotion of patients' rights in Europe. 1994. Copenhagen, WHO Regional Office for Europe.

[3]   Tugend A,.Harris L. Patients' rights in Europe. *Eurohealth* 1997;3:31–3.

[4]   Department of Health. The Patient's Charter. 1992. London, HMSO.

[5]   Farrell, C., Levenson, R., and Snape, D. The Patient's Charter: past and future. 1998. London, King's Fund.

[6]   Dyke, G. The new NHS Charter – a different approach. 1998. London, Department of Health.

[7]   Department of Health. Your guide to the NHS. 2001. London, Department of Health.

[8]   Saltman RB. Patient choice and patient empowerment in northern European health systems: a conceptual framework. *International Journal of Health Services* 1994;24:201–29.

[9]   Bynoe, I. Beyond the Citizen's Charter. 1996. London, Institute for Public Policy Research.

[10] Dabbs, I. At the crossroads: the future of Community Health Councils. Representing the public's interest and citizen involvement in health and health care. 1998. London, School for Social Entrepreneurs.

[11] Pickard S. The future organisation of Community Health Councils. *Social Policy and Administration* 1997;31:274–89.

[12] Rolfe, M., Holden, D., and Lawes, H. Reflecting the public interest - focused, professional. 1998. Bristol, NHS Executive South and West Region.

[13] Hutton W, Commission on the NHS. New life for health. London: Vintage, 2000.

[14] Department of Health. Involving patients and the public in healthcare: response to the listening exercise. www.doh.gov.uk/involving patients . 2001.

[15] Department of Health. Involving patients and the public in healthcare: a discussion document. 2001. London, Department of Health.

[16] Brown I. Patient participation groups in general practice in the National Health Service. *Health Expectations* 1999;2:169–78.

[17] Agass M, Coulter A, Mant D, Fuller A. Patient participation in general practice: who participates? *British Journal of General Practice* 1991;41:198–201.

[18] Wood B. Patient power? Buckingham: Open University Press, 2000.

[19] Department of Health. Local voices: the views of local people in purchasing for health. 1992. London, NHS Management Executive.

[20] Cooper, L., Coote, A., Davies, A., and Jackson, C. Voices off: tackling the democratic deficit in health. 1995. London, Institute for Public Policy Research.

[21] Richardson A. Determining priorities for purchasers: the public response to rationing within the NHS. *Journal of Management in Medicine* 1997;11:222–32.

[22] McIver, S. Healthy debate? An independent evaluation of citizen's juries in health settings. 1998. London, King's Fund.

23   Davies, A., Elizabeth, S., Hanley, B., New, B., and Sang, B. Ordinary wisdom: reflections on an experiment in citizenship and health. 1998. London, King's Fund.

24   Anderson, W., Florin, D., Gillam, S., and Mountford, L. Every voice counts: primary care organisations and public involvement. 2002. London, King's Fund.

25   Daniels N. Justice, fair procedures, and the goals of medicine. *Hastings Center Report* 1996;10–2.

26   Ham C. Tragic choices in health care: lessons from the Child B case. *British Medical Journal* 1999;319:1258–61.

27   Klein, R. and New, B. Two cheers? Reflections on the health of NHS democracy. 1998. London, King's Fund.

7. What can be done in primary care?

I have argued that public expectations are changing and that clinical practice and the organisation of health care delivery must change too. A more active role for the patient and greater public involvement in health policy-making could help to ensure more appropriate treatment and care, improve health outcomes, reduce errors and improve safety, reduce complaints and litigation, raise quality standards, and improve accountability, public understanding and social solidarity. Changes are required at all levels of the system, but primary care professionals have an especially important part to play because they are the first point of contact with the health service and because patients look to them as the primary source of information and advice. As I hope I have demonstrated in the preceding chapters, there is no shortage of ideas about what could be done, and a considerable body of evidence already exists to support its implementation. What is needed now is concerted action by all stakeholders in the system to ensure the potential benefits are realised.

This final chapter summarises the arguments and outlines practical steps that could be taken in primary care to acknowledge and support the patient as an autonomous player in the process of health management and improvement. Primary care teams need to listen to and understand patients' expectations and preferences. They must respect patients' autonomy and acknowledge their role as decision-makers, care managers, evaluators and active citizens. If every primary care team were to adopt the suggested changes, it could trigger a revolution in the way in which people interact with health services.

1. **Understand patients' preferences and expectations**
   The NHS was born in an era when doctors' authority and expertise was revered and their decisions were rarely challenged. There was no need to seek patients' views because doctors knew what was best. This may have felt like a comfortable position for the doctors, but it was not sustainable in the longer term. Attitudes began to change in the 1970s and 80s when the introduction of consumerism and market competition into public services became part of the new political orthodoxy. Markets require active consumers, so patients

were encouraged to take a less passive role and to assert their rights. Although there was resistance to the notion that healthcare could be reduced to anything resembling a series of commercial transactions, ideas about a stronger role for the consumer found a receptive audience among people who were growing increasingly irritated with paternalistic relationships in medical care. In particular women's health groups had drawn attention to the deficiencies of the traditional medical model and its tendency to demean and disempower patients. They emphasised self-education and self-help as a way of redressing the power imbalance between doctors and patients.

Nowadays the fashion for market solutions has waned somewhat, but the challenges to medical dominance are still very much on the agenda. Doctors continue to be held in very high regard by the public, but attitudes and expectations have changed. People expect to be offered choices and want professionals to take account of their preferences. However, medical education still operates under the shadow of the earlier paternalistic era and many doctors have not been trained to listen to patients and take account of their preferences. Time is a scarce commodity in general practice and, since patients often appear comfortable with a directive style, many clinicians see little need for change.

There are lots of reasons why change can seem impractical or undesirable, but these barriers must be overcome. Paternalism is harmful to health because it fosters passivity, sapping self-confidence and undermining people's ability to cope. Paternalistic relationships create and reinforce dependence on health professionals. This in turn breeds resentment on both sides. Clinicians feel their time and skills are being taken up with trivial problems that don't need their input, or social problems which they don't have the resources to tackle. Patients feel disappointed and disillusioned when medical care doesn't live up to their expectations or when treatment isn't as effective as they'd been led to believe. To break this cycle patients must be encouraged to see themselves as partners in the process of health improvement and disease management, with a share in the responsibility for ensuring that health care resources are used as appropriately and efficiently as possible. Failure to do this will lead to further intensification of demand for professional help, resulting in even greater burdens on those working in primary care.

The first step that clinicians in primary care could take to begin the process
of patient empowerment is to understand patients' expectations by actively
listening to them, by giving patients opportunities to ask questions, and by
offering clear and honest answers (Box 1).

Box 1

Listening to individual patients

- Ask patients about their experience of illness and how it and the
  treatment affects their lives.
- Offer opportunities for patients to ask questions and check their
  understanding of the answers.
- Encourage patients with long-term conditions to keep records or diaries
  of their experiences of treatment and review these with them.

Learning to see things through the patient's eyes should be a central part of
professional training and continuing development. This must also include
the views of minority groups and patients from different backgrounds or
cultures. The best way to do this is to actively engage patients in the process
of training health professionals. There are a number of ways primary care
teams and those responsible for organising professional development could
tackle this (Box 2).

Box 2

Learning from patients

- Organise focus groups with specific groups of patients or carers
  (e.g. those with chronic diseases, those caring for people recovering
  from stroke, patients from ethnic minorities, asylum seekers, etc.) to
  learn more about their experiences and how the practice or Primary
  Care Trust can meet their specific needs.
- Learn about the needs, values and illness perceptions of people from
  minority ethnic groups (cultural competence training).
- Learn more about the needs of people with disabilities (disability
  awareness training)
- Use videos of patients talking about their experience of illness and
  treatment in educational programmes for staff and trainees.

Building on an understanding of the patient's perspective, primary care clinicians can do a great deal to promote realistic expectations. Sick people need empathy, support and reassurance, but they also need honest information about their condition and the treatment options. Most patients want to be able to trust the health professionals they consult, but this does not mean they want to be deceived about the nature of their illness or the risks and potential harms of medical intervention. Trust is very important, but it does not equate to blind faith. Most people want to know the full story, bad news as well as good. They need information about illness and treatments and clear explanations of the nature of clinical evidence and its interpretation. In particular clinicians should be honest with patients about what can and what cannot be done to treat illness or alleviate suffering. They should also acknowledge uncertainty and be willing to say when they don't know the answer (Box 3).

Box 3

Honest communication

- When you don't know the best course of action, be willing to admit it.
- If there's no effective treatment for a patient's problem, say so.
- Use graphics, computer programmes and other techniques to explain risk and outcome probabilities.
- Give patients non-alarmist information about medicine side-effects.
- Provide information on what patients can do to help themselves.
- Educate patients about how to prevent illness and prevent recurrence.

2. **Patient as decision-maker**

Patients need access to information if they are to participate in decisions about their care. Good quality information materials can greatly assist clinicians in their efforts to improve communication with patients and encourage their active involvement. There is a great deal of unreliable information about, but better designed, more reliable information tools are increasingly becoming available and primary care staff should aim to help their patients access them. The National Electronic Library for Health is a useful resource, NHS Direct Online provides web-based access to information about diseases and treatments, the Doctor Patient Partnership has published a series of guides, and various commercial information providers and some voluntary groups have developed useful packages. Much of this material still has an old-fashioned feel, often being too didactic and simplistic, but the choice and quality of patient information is improving rapidly.

Leaflets, charts or booklets can be very useful, as can audio or video tapes, but the internet greatly increases the potential for patient education and the explosion of health web sites shows no sign of slowing down. Sorting out the wheat from the chaff in this information feast is not easy, but there are various guides and quality assessment tools available to help. Primary care staff should be aware of what is available and ready to help their patients find the most reliable information. Many patients will not have access to the internet at home or even at work, but computers with internet access could be made available in general practices and other health facilities for use by patients.

Many clinicians will object that they do not have time to carry out the additional tasks of informing and educating. In the long run there is no reason to think that empowered patients will demand more time from individual clinicians, indeed demand for professional help might reduce. But the burden does not have to fall solely on the GP or nurse practitioner. Trained information staff could take some of the load and other health professionals, for example, pharmacists, could have an important role to play. Better team-working and better use of information technology could free up professional time to meet patients' information needs more efficiently than relying on the GP as the sole information source.

What is needed is a new cadre of 'information brokers' who can help people find, interpret and use health information. Most patients currently see their GPs as the first port of call when they want information about their health, but GPs do not always have the necessary skills in information retrieval to do a good job. NHS Direct has a role to play here, but more direct, personal help will be needed by many patients. It wouldn't cost a great deal to appoint a small team of health information staff to work in each Primary Care Trust. They would need expertise in information sources and how to access them and well-developed skills in critical appraisal, but essentially two or three trained information staff and a computer with internet access is all that is required. Patients could consult the information broker instead of their GP if information is all they require, or they could be referred to them by the GP or nurse practitioner for more detailed information searching following a consultation. Similar information teams could work in Acute Trusts and Mental Health Trusts to help patients access the information they need. This relatively small investment could relieve clinicians of a considerable burden on their time. Information could be seen as part of a therapeutic package, with clinicians 'prescribing' information in the same way they might prescribe medicines (Box 4).

Box 4

Information for patients

- Establish a library of good quality patient information materials.
- Research information sources on the web so you can advise patients about where to look for relevant information.
- Make a computer in the practice available for patients to search the web for health information.
- Publicise reliable information sources such as the National Electronic Library for Health, NHS Direct, etc.
- Encourage the Primary Care Trust to employ specialist staff to act as information brokers.

As patients become more knowledgeable, clinicians will find they need to devote more time to explaining and negotiating. Some will feel threatened by these changes that seem to challenge their authority. They may fear that their role is being reduced to that of facilitator rather than decision maker, devaluing their clinical expertise and their status. But the clock cannot be turned back. As co-producers of their own health patients have to be provided with the means to make rational decisions about their health care. The professional's role is to support this process. This need not be seen as undermining the clinician's role. On the contrary, it could make it more satisfying and productive. Patients who are well-informed about prognosis and treatment options are more likely to adhere to treatments, leading to better health outcomes. They are also less likely to accept ineffective or risky procedures.

Much has been written about the skills necessary to involve patients in shared decisions about their care. Shared decision-making demands excellent communication skills and many clinicians will require extra training to develop these. Observation of consultation processes has demonstrated that achieving a partnership approach is more difficult than it sounds and requires the development of a new set of competences (Box 5). Nevertheless, the studies show that expending the effort to engage patients in this way can be very worthwhile. Professional organisations should revise their curricula so that communication skills are given greater priority. The principles of shared decision-making, concordance in medicine-taking and strategies to promote self-management should feature prominently in the curriculum, together with development of the skills to explain probability, risk and uncertainty.

In addition public money should be made available to fund the development of a suite of evidence-based decision aids for patients and make these available in every general practice. This would not be difficult or especially expensive, and it is likely to prove cost-effective since patients given full information and the opportunity to choose tend to opt for the least risky, and often cheaper, alternative. As we saw in chapter 3, many patient decision aids have been developed and tested, but few have been made generally available. Decision aids developed in the USA or Canada would be relatively easy to adapt for UK use and further development of new materials to support informed choice could be modelled along the same lines.

Box 5

Sharing treatment decisions

- Keep a collection of paper-based decision aids and/or a list of internet addresses for web-based decision aids and refer patients to these.
- Involve patients in defining and clarifying the problem or diagnosis.
- Explore their ideas, fears and preferences.
- Provide information about treatment options and outcomes and discuss these.
- Ask patients about their preferred level of involvement in decisions.
- Elicit patient's treatment preferences using a decision aid where feasible.
- Check patient's views and preferred course of action.
- Find out what patients feel about taking medicines before writing a prescription.
- If a specialist referral is indicated, discuss the goals of this with the patient.

3. **Patient as care manager**

People who have long-term conditions already play an important role in managing their own care. The development of technologies for self-monitoring physiological status and clinical indicators, for example ambulatory blood pressure monitors, cholesterol testing kits, and blood glucose meters, is hastening the trend towards self-management of chronic diseases. Increasingly patients will be able to coordinate and monitor their own care, under the guidance of health professionals. This role needs to be recognised and supported by providing access to relevant information and educational programmes (Box 6).

Patients with chronic diseases need to learn how to interpret symptoms and changes in their condition. They need strategies for coping with physical and emotional problems caused by their illness and, if they are likely to need specialist help and support, they need to know where to find this and how to access it. Care plans should be developed and agreed with the patient, taking account of their specific situation and ability to cope with or without help. Many will continue to depend on family or other informal carers for support. Primary care staff should be aware of carers' needs and work with them to ensure that care plans take account of the patient's and carer's social situation.

Patients who know what to expect can check on appropriate performance of clinical tasks. They can also ensure that medicines and other treatments are taken safely and appropriately. Clinical guidelines should be made available to patients so they can monitor their own care and ensure that everything that could be done is being done. Encouraging patients to be alert to deviations from agreed protocols could help to reduce adverse events and promote safety.

As was described in chapter 4, training materials and courses to support self-care and self-management of chronic diseases have been developed by academics and voluntary groups. Work is currently under way to encourage further dissemination of these ideas and training opportunities through the auspices of the Department of Health-funded Expert Patient programme. Since chronic disease management constitutes the major responsibility of general practice, primary care professionals should be involved in shaping and developing this programme and encouraging their patients to participate.

Box 6

Support for self-management

- Involve patients in developing care plans and offer choices wherever possible.
- Give patients copies of clinical guidelines – for example, the National Institute for Clinical Excellence publishes patient versions of its guidelines.
- Involve patients in reviewing their medication.
- Put patients in touch with self-help groups and other sources of information about chronic disease.
- Where appropriate refer patients to self-management training programmes.
- Involve carers and inform them about support services.

It is extraordinary that up until quite recently it was seen as unexceptional that records kept by health professionals should not be available to the person to whom they are most relevant, i.e. the patient. Patients have a right to know what is being communicated about them between professionals and they should be encouraged to read their notes. As long as they have been kept fully in the picture, these should not be unduly alarming. Patients could be encouraged to append their own comments to the records and to draw attention to any errors or omissions. They should also be given copies of referral letters and test results as a matter of routine (Box 7). When the transition to electronic health records is finally complete, these could be stored on secure websites, with access controlled by patients themselves via smart cards. In the meantime, patients should be encouraged to read and check their medical records, including those stored on computers.

Box 7

Access to medical records

- Allow patients access to their records and encourage them to review them, add to them and correct any errors.
- Where appropriate use shared care cards which can be held by the patient.

- Give patients copies of referral letters and test results and be ready to explain these.
- If the practice uses electronic records, make arrangements for patients to access these via terminals in the practice.

Even though patients now have a legal right to look at their records, barriers are often placed in the way to prevent them doing so. Some practices even charge patients for access to their medical notes. This situation should not be allowed to continue since it casts the patient as the dependent object of care, rather than as an active coordinator of services.

4. **Patient as evaluator**

It makes sense to identify and tackle problems before they become serious issues. The best way to do this in healthcare is to seek feedback from patients. Patients' views on the quality of care they have received should be a key part of any performance assessment system. Regular, systematic patient surveys can be used alongside morbidity and mortality reviews to audit performance and set benchmarks and standards. Using the results of patient surveys to inform quality improvement programmes is a powerful way of reorienting efforts towards more patient-centred approaches to healthcare delivery (Box 8).

Box 8

Patient feedback and quality assessment

- Organise regular patient surveys and use the findings to set priorities for quality improvement.
- Use brief questionnaires after consultations to elicit patients' views on communication and interpersonal skills.
- Organise a patient participation group and enlist their help in reviewing practice organisation and suggesting improvements.
- Review disabled access – involve disabled people.
- Publicise and review the complaints procedure.
- Give patients feedback on any changes made.

The evidence suggests that patients are most likely to be concerned about access and waiting times, having a choice of who to consult, having sufficient information, space and time to explain their needs and concerns, and being treated with respect and dignity by staff. There is much that could be done to ensure these requirements are met (Box 9).

Box 9

Improving patients experience within the practice

- Ensure patients are given sufficient privacy, including in the reception area.
- Arrange customer care training for reception staff and where appropriate involve patients in this.
- Allow patients to choose which practitioner they wish to consult.
- Offer direct appointments with nurses, counsellors and other staff.
- Arrange consultation skills training for all staff, not just doctors, and use patient feedback to monitor the outcome.
- Monitor patient flows and ask receptionists to keep a note of how long patients are kept waiting.
- Make time available during the day for telephone or email consultations.

As referrers and commissioners of secondary care, primary care staff and PCTs can do a great deal to improve patients' experience in hospital. By involving patients in referral decisions and ensuring that selection of provider is informed by evidence on the quality of care, it should be possible to direct patients to the most appropriate place and, where necessary, exert influence on secondary care providers if improvements are required (Box 10). It is also important to discuss and agree with the patient the reason for referral to a specialist and to communicate this clearly to the specialist when making the referral. All parties are then better placed to evaluate the outcome and to determine whether the agreed objectives have been achieved.

Information about waiting times and the quality of health services is available through the Department of Health's national performance assessment framework and the performance indicators that are published on a regular basis in the press, but these league tables are not easy for the layman to comprehend or use without help. It has been left to a commercial company,

Dr Foster, to provide information on local services specifically designed for the public. Their healthcare guides and website are better designed than those published by the Department of Health and they are becoming quite popular, although there has been some criticism of the reliability of the information they contain. The information should be validated by an independent source, and, assuming it is found to be reliable, all GPs and primary care staff should be familiar with it so they can discuss it with their patients and use the information when making referral decisions.

Box 10

Improving patients' experience of secondary care

- Ensure that performance information can be accessed and understood by practice staff and patients.
- Review performance indicators with patients and offer referral choices.
- Check convenience to patient of referral location and timing.
- Agree with the patient on the reason for referral and communicate this to the specialist.
- Monitor the length of time patients are waiting for outpatient consultations or inpatient admission.

5. **Patient as active citizen**

No health system can function long without public support. The desire to promote public involvement is borne out of the difficulties faced by governments and health authorities struggling with the need to control health care costs while satisfying raised public expectations. As more and more effective but costly treatments are developed, policy-makers must try to ensure that the gap between expectations and supply in health care does not run out of control. By encouraging patients and citizens to play a more active role in health care and health improvement, they hope to promote appropriate use of cost-effective services, but, even more importantly, this would appear to be the best way to shore up social solidarity, the essential underpinning of a sustainable health system. Systems based on exclusion, inequity and secrecy do not have a future. Public involvement in, and democratic accountability for, decisions about healthcare priorities, including decisions about what is affordable out of public resources, will become more and more essential. Public ignorance of the issues breeds unrealistic aspirations and inappropriately simplistic political responses.

Primary care professionals cannot be expected to hold sole responsibility for promoting realistic expectations, but they have an important role to play in helping people to understand the limitations of medical care (Box 13). Public education is required to encourage people to appraise health information critically and to help them understand the concepts of probability and risk and how to cope with uncertainty. Ideally this should start in schools, but it could also be incorporated into occupational training schemes and public education via the media. When major public health issues arise, for example, the BSE crisis or the MMR scare, it is important that the public is given the full facts right at the start, instead of hoping that bland reassurances will be sufficient. People are increasingly sceptical and mistrustful of government information, but they do still place considerable trust in health professionals. Since patients often turn to their GP for advice, primary care staff need to be brought into the loop at the beginning so they can help explain the issue to worried patients (Box 11).

Box 11

Public education about health and healthcare

- Keep informed about media health scares and about the facts behind the stories so you can answer patients' queries.
- Be willing to talk to journalists and help the media publish accurate information.
- Be aware of commercial promotion and its effects on the demand for healthcare and encourage a sceptical approach.
- Try to keep informed about epidemiological evidence on disease risk factors and systematic reviews on treatment efficacy and use this knowledge in discussions with patients.

Even though healthcare in the NHS is largely free at the point of use, as current or past taxpayers the patients who use the service are also paying for it. As funders they want to feel confident that their money is well spent. Public accountability and transparent procedures are crucial at both national and local levels, and should be embedded in the governance of Primary Care Trusts. Professionals and officials will have to adapt their style to accommodate this more open approach.

Current initiatives to involve patient representatives in decision-making bodies are very welcome, but these lay representatives will need support and training if they are to play an influential role. It is important to work with organised patient and community groups, but their views must be balanced by those of non-activists whose views must be actively sought out. Just as decision making at the one-to-one level of the clinical consultation should take account of the principles of shared decision making, so must those responsible for allocating health care resources seek legitimacy by involving the public and ensuring that the basis for their decisions is transparent and open to challenge if necessary.

Primary Care Trusts have an important role as commissioners of health services. They have the task of ensuring that individual clinical decisions fit within the wider context of resource availability and public priorities. This is extremely difficult since the potential for medical technologies to achieve beneficial effects for larger numbers of people with a wider range of conditions and ailments is increasing faster than the public's willingness to pay for them. Patient choice cannot be divorced from its societal context and when individual expectations clash with population priorities there must be a mechanism for resolving the conflict. The challenge is to harness its potential to improve the effectiveness of medical care, while ensuring that it does not undermine the principles of solidarity and fairness that underpin public confidence in health care systems. The balancing act of individual needs versus population requirements cannot be left to 'experts' alone. Patients and citizens need to understand the choices confronting policy-makers and need to be involved in determining priorities and trade-offs. As we saw in chapter 6, various techniques for identifying citizens' views on health care priorities have been developed and Primary Care Trusts could use these to consult local citizens (Box 12).

Box 12

Engaging the public in policy decisions

- Hold meetings in public wherever possible and publish agendas and minutes.
- Use formal techniques, such as citizen's juries or patient forums, to consult local people on priorities.
- Be prepared to explain the reasons for unpopular decisions (e.g. closure of services) and establish a formal process of appeal.
- Offer training to lay representatives on committees.
- Work with local voluntary organisations and patient and community groups.
- Actively seek the views of minority groups and people who do not belong to patient or community organisations.
- Ensure that local people are kept informed of their rights and responsibilities.

Conclusions

It has become commonplace to play lip service to the need for patient and public involvement in healthcare, but the reality doesn't match the rhetoric at present. Many public involvement initiatives are little more than window dressing. Involving a few token patients on committees is relatively easy to do, but it does nothing to tackle the heart of the problem, which is that healthcare delivery is still steeped in paternalism. The really important changes need to occur at the level of individual interactions between patients and health professionals.

We might expect this type of cultural change to occur slowly, but the health system is at risk if it continues to resist adaptation to changes in public expectations. Some critics see attempts to promote a more patient-centred approach as peripheral to the serious business of treatment and care, an unnecessary and burdensome addition to the long list of demands made on health professionals. Others dismiss it as mere political correctness, a temporary fashion that can be ignored. Yet others fear it will be too costly, believing that recognising patients' autonomy and taking account of their preferences will increase the demand for scarce resources to unsustainable levels.

In this monograph I have tried to show that these objections miss the point altogether. Far from being peripheral, the development of a more active role for the patient and the citizen will be fundamental to securing the future of public healthcare. It is the only way to ensure its affordability, acceptability and sustainability over the long term. Healthcare is too important to leave in the hands of professionals alone and anyway it is in their interest to ensure that the responsibility is shared. I hope those working in primary care will accept the challenge to lead the way in developing active partnerships with the patients they serve.